ASPECTS OF GREEK AND ROMAN LIFE

General Editor: H. H. Scullard

★ ★ ★

ROMAN MEDICINE

John Scarborough

ROMAN MEDICINE

John Scarborough

CORNELL UNIVERSITY PRESS
ITHACA, NEW YORK

First published 1969

Standard Book Number: 8014–0525–4

Library of Congress Catalog Card Number: 72–81596

PRINTED IN ENGLAND

CONTENTS

6   CONTENTS

LIST OF ILLUSTRATIONS

PLATES

FIGURES

PREFACE

THIS STUDY is not intended as a technical treatise on the details of Roman medicine. Rather it examines the Roman view of medicine, and draws a few conclusions on the nature of medicine in the Roman world. Since the appearance of Sir Clifford Allbutt's *Greek Medicine in Rome* (London, 1921), there has been no work putting Roman medicine and its development before the modern reader. Studies which have appeared normally investigate aspects of the 'scientific application' practised in medicine among the Romans. Such studies greatly enrich our knowledge of the ancient world, and how the ancients conceived the natural world, but very often modern terminologies superimpose themselves upon ancient definitions. For medicine as it existed among the Greeks and Romans, one of the basic problems is simply conceptualization, that is just *how* close were *their* concepts to ours. We all work within a given frame of reference, but hopefully, when we study a culture which is both alien and similar, we must beware of preconceptions which warp the historical picture to suit our own tastes.

For many of the ideas presented in *Roman Medicine*, I must first admit my great debt to the writings of Ludwig Edelstein, one of the great scholars in ancient medicine it was my privilege to read and ponder. I never met Professor Edelstein, but felt many common bonds through fascination about ancient medicine. He was an uncompromising iconoclast in the destruction of outmoded ideas of the ancient world. In his work, he continually warned that we must not assume our concept of the normal in medicine was necessarily that of the ancients, whatever their achievement. Proof of such arguments came from Keith Hopkins and his work on the problem of contraception in the Roman Empire. Here, as Hopkins amply indicates, the Romans did practise what *we* call contraception, but often did not think of it as prevention.

Greek medicine gave the great inspiration of the rationalization of disease, but never sought to put the study of medicine above the reach of the educated man. The development of scholarly medicine in the Hellenistic world showed a tendency to specialize, but not always in the exploration of new ideas. With the startling exceptions of Erasistratus and Herophilus, the Alexandrian Museum stood as a centre of consolidation and commentary in scholarly efforts, including medicine. As Hellenistic medicine spread throughout the Roman world, and collided with Roman native medicine, we find borrowing and adaptation in both methods. Hellenistic medicine, practised among the Romans by physicians schooled in the concepts of Hippocrates, Praxagoras, and their successors, never lost its predilection for the general and spoke with the authority of philosophy. The Romans, on their part, remained sceptical, and valued their own tradition of medicine well expressed in Cato, Celsus and Varro. Galen summed the total of ancient medicine in his huge corpus, and it contains Roman practical outlooks as well as the philosophical learning typical of the Galenic ideal of the philosopher-physician. Celsus' version of the Roman *medicus-pater familias* had many links with Hellenistic medicine, but Celsus adapted when he thought Hellenistic ideas gave better answers to Roman practical questions.

Celsus recognized various shades of opinion among his Hellenistic predecessors, and modern students of Roman medicine usually overlabel these 'schools', or 'sects'. In the following study, I will put 'school' or 'sect' in quotations to indicate my feeling that too much distinction between the various shades of interpretation in Hellenistic and Roman medicine is often unwarranted. If the term 'school' is used properly, philosophical differences—that is differing approaches to the theory of medicine—are what Galen and Celsus mean as they speak of 'those of opposing "sects" '.

To analyse Roman medicine in its proper light, we must consider such matters as education, the social matrix, and religion. In the history of science in general, one needs to recall that 'scientists' of whatever age are men of faith. In the early history of Roman medicine, the Roman version of 'doctor' also meant 'priest', and subjective concepts followed observation of nature. Roman ideas of the natural world were based on practical considerations, and before the introduction of theoretical medicine from the Hellenistic world, Roman needs on the farm formed the core of immediate knowledge of medical treatment. Nevertheless, we can consider the Roman farmer in the early period a scientist, if we are careful not to impose twentieth-century analogies upon his ideals. Theoretical matters had little place in Roman agriculture, but his manner of handling supernatural things gave the early Roman the conviction that his view of the universe was essentially correct. We may term the early period of Roman medicine religious, and the religious opinion formed the foundation of positive action. Such is the way of scientists, whatever their age or origin. With this consideration in mind, there seems to be little separating the scientist from the so-called layman with the exception that the scientist occasionally refuses to admit the ravages of chance. The Roman attitude towards theory is similar to the question put by Alice to the Dodo, 'What is a Caucus-Race?' with the Dodo's reply, 'the best way to explain it is to do it.'

For the reader who may be interested in a more technical consideration of Roman medicine, Galen and Celsus have been translated into English, and their writing on surgery, drugs, some aspects of anatomy and the rest can be read by anyone. A word of caution must accompany this recommendation. Often translators are forced to extrapolate from modern terms and sometimes this can lead to misrepresentation of the Latin or Greek involved. The whole problem of medicine among the Romans should invite learned curiosity, especially that of the professional classicist or ancient historian, who may find many aspects of my *Roman Medicine* subjects for discussion. If I stimulate interest in a neglected topic of major importance, I will feel the book has succeeded in its basic purpose.

Many individuals have contributed their effort and time in aiding the composition of this book. I especially wish to express my thanks to Professor Chester Starr of the University of Illinois, who read a draft and offered many valuable comments on its composition and content. Professor Raymond Stearns provided the first stimulus of interest in the problems of the history of medicine, and it is to him I owe an unflagging fascination for an often difficult area. The idea for a study of Roman medicine was first formulated while I was a medical student at the University of Kansas, where I enjoyed the acquaintance of Professor L. R. C. Agnew. I owe special thanks to the untiring help of the staff of the University of Illinois Classics Library, as well as to the generosity of the librarians at the University of Kentucky Medical Center. I was privileged to work for short periods in the Logan Clendening Library in Kansas City, Kansas, and the Wellcome Institute of the History of Medicine, London, where I received encouragement and assistance. I am indebted to the cordial staff of the Museum of Antiquities, Amman, Jordan, for permission to make photographs and sketches of numerous Greco-Roman objects throwing valuable light on medicine. To my wife, Ginger, I owe the ultimate gratitude of listening to my ideas, and then unweaving them to make sense for the non-classical reader.

Lexington, Kentucky,
    December, 1968

CHAPTER I

THE BEGINNINGS OF ROMAN MEDICINE

MISTS OF LEGEND and uncertainty surround Rome's origins but archaeological research in the twentieth century has begun to give light to an important and complex period. The complicated heritage of Roman customs and the sources for the Roman frame of reference are emerging in dim outline.[1] Archaeological and linguistic evidence blend to indicate the unique characteristics Rome achieved at the crossroads of early Italy. Roman medical concepts ultimately stemmed from these inheritances, based solidly upon agriculture and its accompanying religious practices.

Early Rome and its religious outlook determined the perception of healing. The Romans felt 'the gods were supreme lords and governors of all things and events were directed by their influence, wisdom, and divine power.'[2] Misfortunes were simply punishment for neglect or offence, and took the expressed form of some divinity or divine force. Beneath the sophisticated words of Cicero was the Roman feeling that the forces of nature, which were the results of divine will, were mysterious and could be but placated, not understood.[3] Conceptualization of these forces in human form came only after the Etruscans had adapted for themselves Greek concepts. Since Rome was an Etruscan city for a time during the seventh and sixth centuries BC, Roman ideas of the primitive *numina* were infused with the Greco-Etruscan anthropomorphism. None the less, the Roman gods and goddesses, particularly those of the countryside, remained but one short step from the earlier native Italic views. Some force ruled all human actions,[4] and a spirit of some kind was assumed for everything that existed.

The men, the state, the family pantry, all had their counterpart of nature's actions in the spiritual world.[5] After 500 BC, the great gods and goddesses came to describe larger spheres spoken of in abstraction, and there were gods on a lesser plane as well as countless *numina*, which might or might not be named. Each had a function with a defined activity, seen in the world of nature and men. Most *numina* were vague, hazily outlined forces, which had lives of their own, but were not conceived of in a personal fashion. Others received transparent names, indicating their action, probably due to priestly invention, and many of these are found in surviving sacred litanies.[6]

Early Roman medical concepts were embodied in the prevailing religion of the countryside. Any person who had to perform a delicate task recognized that he could not originate the power to do his deed, but could, with proper ceremonies, direct the *numen* which would give a desired result. Apparently the early Romans felt a given instrument used for a specific job *was* the *numen* in question. The shrine of Mars contained spears which were thought to be Mars, that is the spears *were* Mars. Later Romans were puzzled by this and thought of them as the spears of Mars, showing the emergence of anthropomorphic symbolism.[7] The *numina* exhibited themselves in highly specialized ways, as in possible relief from discomfort or disease.

Disease was a force of divine displeasure the Romans experienced from time to time. They based their response to the ravages of plague upon the impersonal concept of wrath from an unknown source for unknown reasons. The Senate called upon the people to pray to the gods, 'to supplicate with their wives and children'.[8] Here we note the lack of good historical record for early visitations of pestilence, since Livy takes a bare fact and lets his imagination fill the gaps. Livy's guess is probable as he gives a graphic picture of widespread public prayer.[9] Other authors use similar phrases to describe such instances,[10] and Livy makes clear the religious connection in his choice of words reminiscent of religious phraseology.[11] Possibly the diseases encountered by the early Romans were malaria, typhus, and anthrax, or a combination of several pestilences.[12] Since the diseases eventually went away, the Romans assumed they had managed to perform the correct actions of contrition, although they did not attempt to understand the disease or its recession. Livy adds his own explanation to his sparse sources on the return of health to Rome, 'whether it came from the obtained favour of the gods, or the unhealthy part of the year was over.'[13]

Roman native medicine had a strong tradition often noted in our sources. The Romans thought physicians did not exist in their early history, but supposed the Romans of old practised medicine in general terms.[14] Upon casual reading of Pliny and Cato the Elder, the narrative seems to abound with old wives' tales which might support the assertion that early Roman medicine consisted solely of 'folk' traditions.[15] Yet the modern concept of magic and religion differs markedly from that of the ancient world.[16] Possibly the term 'magical-rational' is suitable for instinctive medicine developed in primitive societies.[17] The medical outlook of the Romans in the first two centuries of the Republic fits this pattern, as they chose to treat themselves and their families rather than develop a theoretical medicine as had the Greeks.[18] Early Roman medicine should be described as popular or quasi-religious, rather than irrational.

An excellent example of the religious, yet semi-rational tendency of early Roman medicine is found in the collection of Aulus Gellius. Gellius borrows matter from Varro and tells us how the Romans in the early days set up altars to the spirits of natural and unnatural births.

> Thus when it happened that [the children in the womb] were turned upon their feet contrary to nature, women gave birth with greater difficulty since their arms are extended. To avoid this danger, altars were set up in Rome to the two Carmentes. One was named Postverta,[19] and the other Prorsa.[20] They were designated by natural and unnatural birth and the power therein.[21]

The tradition of Roman religion was powerful. Carmenta was a goddess of birth, and her festival, the Carmentalia, was observed

B

on January 11 and 15. Probably the Roman custom preserved the
Carmentes as deified symbols of earlier midwives, or 'wise
women' who were called upon to assist in births.[22]

Although a kind of rationality was characteristic of early
Roman medicine, our sources consider only remedies. Diagnosis,
prognosis, and regimen were not taken into significant consideration. This pattern is unusual, since in the normal development of
popular medicine in uncivilized tribes, these matters receive much
emphasis.[23] Religious cures were rare but magical treatment was
common. Cato records a prayer to Mars Silvanus, for the continued health of cattle, which will have its desired effect even
when uttered by a slave.[24] Later Cato gives an offering with a
prayer to Jupiter Dapalis for the health of cattle.[25] The account
contains other prayers with offerings. Similar is Cato's formula
for the warding of sickness from his household.

> Father Mars, I entreat and beg you . . . to keep at bay, repulse,
> and take away disease, known and arcane . . . and to give
> health to me, my house, and my household.[26]

> Present your little heap of offering cakes to Janus saying,
> 'Father Janus, offering these cakes to you, I contritely beseech
> you to be merciful and kind to me and my children, my
> house, and my household.'[27]

The title 'father' further indicates how the Romans conceived
of the power of actions, and how sometimes honorific titles were
bestowed on these powers, the most common being 'father' and
'mother' words. There is no etymological connection here with
bearing or begetting children, but they suggested to the Roman
the meaning of religious and legal power.[28] Horace tells how a
mother of a child with fever that occurs every four days prays to
Jupiter to cure him. If the blessing was performed, the child stood
naked in the Tiber on the following feast day.[29]

Pliny the Elder glances back into an earlier era and sees Cato the
Elder practising medicine in the ancient, unsophisticated mould.
According to Pliny, Cato's medicine was effective since he
lived to a ripe old age of 85. Cato prolonged his own life and the

lives of his family by what Pliny classifies as 'native' remedies. The
early Romans, as Pliny records them, did not ignore medicine, but
condemned the 'art of medicine, mainly because they refused to
give payment to profiteers to preserve their lives'.[30] The medicine
Pliny sees in Cato's writing is similar to that of the midwives
called upon to help in births, and reminds one of the *medicus* or
obstetrix who appears in interpretations of the *Lex Aquilia* of the
third century BC.[31] The term *medicus* took its origin within the
framework of the early practices of medicine on the farm. Of the
three chapters of the law which are extant, two show that damage
to property was the primary concern.[32] The farm is the scene of
the problem, and later interpretations put the *medicus* and the
obstetrix as well as the *tonsor* into this context.[33] The matrix of the
early law suggests the Romans recognized persons who professed
to know of such matters, but they were of the lower social ranks.

The *pater familias* was the dispenser of remedies of his household,
and Cato drew up a list of medicines.[34] He felt his knowledge of
the farm and its needs qualified him to deal with matters of health.
Characteristic of early Roman medicine was a reliance upon one
or two remedies. Unwashed wool, according to the early traditions, dipped into a mixture of pounded rue[35] and fat, was good
for bruises and swellings. Wool and honey rubbed on the gums
made the breath pleasing. A bleeding nose could be cured by the
insertion of wool and rose oil. Ram's wool, washed in cold water
and soaked in oil, was used to soothe uterine inflammations, and
if fumigation were added, reduced the problems of prolapsus.[36]
Wool dipped into a mixture of oil, sulphur, vinegar, pitch, and
soda cured lumbago.[37] Pliny continues his list of remedies taking
up the various combinations of suint,[38] describing eggs and combinations with honey and the like, reviewing medicaments from
snakes, chickens, insects, birds of all kinds, and so on. Pliny inter-
sperses early Italian traditions with 'modern' ideas, that is those
prescribed by the Greeks and others.[39] Cato's cure-all is cabbage.[40]
Pliny adds the 'early Romans gave wool awesome powers'.[41] con-
firming the religious-agricultural context of early remedies.

Cato's recipes indicate how the Roman attempted to include as
much as possible as he prescribed.

If you have reason to fear sickness, give the oxen before they get sick the following remedy: 3 grains of salt, 3 laurel leaves, 3 leek leaves, 3 spikes of leek, 3 of garlic, 3 grains of incense, 3 plants of Sabine herb, 3 leaves of rue, 3 stalks of bryony, 3 white beans, 3 live coals, and 3 pints of wine. You must gather, macerate, and administer all these while standing, and he who administers the remedy must be fasting. Administer to each ox for three days, and divide it in such a way that when you have administered three doses to each, you have used it all. See to it that the ox and the one who administers are both standing, and use a wooden vessel.[42]

Magical connotation is clear from the continual use of three this or that. Other than the bay leaves, bryony, rue, and live coals, the remedy consists of foodstuffs. The live coals suggest a fever extinguished by the wine. Possibly the standing position is a remnant of psychological factors pointing to an earlier time of a medicine man. The wooden bowl shows the recipe to be an ancient one.[43]

Magical remedies sometimes took the form of chants, whose meaning had become lost like various of the early religious formulae.[44] The agricultural surrounding is clear but religious ties had become obscured by Cato's day. In one formula, dislocation was cured by a charm made from a long green reed, split in the middle, and held to the patient's hip (or wherever the injury occurred). The chants 'motas uaeta daries dardares astatares dissunapiter' and 'haut haut istasis tarsis ardannabout dannaustra' were repeated as the cure was applied.[45] The power in the procedure was couched in the words of the chants, which appear to be nonsense interspersed with Latin syllables. The healing-*numen* originally was thought to exist in the words of the phrases and the symbols of healing, the meaning and significance of which had been forgotten by the time of Cato. Power sifted from the unknown sounds and was accompanied by symbolic action, performed over the patient: the half-reeds showing the fracture has healed. Symbolism from an earlier age gave Cato's prescriptions their effectiveness. After taking a concoction of pomegranate

blossoms, old wine, fennel root, incense, honey and wild mar-
joram for dyspepsia, stomach worms and tapeworms, the patient
had to climb a pillar and jump down ten times.[46]

The Romans inherited some of their ideas of medicine and
anatomy from the Etruscans and adapted them to the practice of
the official state religion.[47] Frequent traces appear in the well-
known Roman practices of divination and augury.[48] The Romans
themselves were perfectly aware of the Etruscan overlay in many
of their activities.[49] Recent archaeological research indicates the
Romans also inherited some of their practice of sanitary architecture from the Etruscans.[50] Votive remains show heavy Etruscan
influence upon early Roman concepts of internal human anatomical features. The rib cage, liver and lower viscera are reproduced in Etruscan and Roman votives with relative fidelity, in the
same manner as are votives of animal entrails. They probably
represent 'normal anatomy' as thought of by the Etrusco-Roman
sculptors of the period to 200 BC,[51] and have direct connection
with the practice of divination.

Since there is little reliable Etruscan evidence for haruspication,
we must cautiously look at near-eastern parallels to gain a general
idea of what was involved in the art of reading livers and its
relationship to medicine. There are problems in this approach, as
indicated by the famous bronze liver found at Piacenza around
1877. It is the subject of much learned argument as to its function
and origin, and shows a different method of hepatoscopy than the
system observed in the near east.[52] The practice of hepatoscopy
was an ancient one, going back to the era of Sargon I.[53] Apparently there was an extensive literature on the methods of liver
reading, and illustrations of tablets exist showing liver anomalies
as well as texts written on models of the liver.[54]

In the Near East, the basic theory behind the value associated
with liver examination was that once an animal had been sacrificed to a god, he identified himself with the spirit of the animal.
The god's wishes would be reflected in the internal organs, especially the liver, which was thought to be the home of the soul and
the centre of life.[55] Complicated ceremonies surrounded the consultation of the liver oracle.[56] After a question was put down in

writing, the tablet was placed at the foot of the god. Then the animal, usually a sheep, was slaughtered and the abdominal cavity opened by a priest who specialized in reading livers (the Etruscan *haruspex*), and he examined the liver and intestines *in situ*. After the priest had inspected the place which the liver had formerly occupied in the abdomen and had cut out the liver, he examined with minute care the whole liver, the left and right lobes, the square lobe, the lobus caudatus, processus capillaris and processus pyramidalis, the gall bladder and ducts, the blood and lymph vessels connected to the liver.[57] Texts were composed and organized after the various parts of the liver.[58] Most of the texts show that the oracle and its elaborate ceremonial were summoned in matters of state, but other surviving examples prove that health and disease were considered.[59]

> If the processus pyramidalis is normal, he who brings the sacrifice will be in good health and he will live a long time.

> . . . if the ductus hepaticus falls to the right the sick will live but will not accomplish his desire.[60]

Many of these practices undoubtedly were carried into Italy, and, in an altered form which is yet unclear, formed a part of the Etruscan art of liver reading. Our view of these ceremonies as we can identify them in Assyria and Babylonia cannot be used to explain Etruscan divination, but we can gain some idea of the original concepts as they emerged from the ancient near east. Such medical concepts, which became fused with Roman ideas, probably had their beginnings in the religious ceremonial surrounding the examination of sacrificed animals. There is, however, some indication that the Etruscans had surgeons and dentists who were well-respected long before the influx of Greek practitioners.[61] The remains of medical instruments from the period suggest something of Near-Eastern qualities and resemble many of the tools from Asia Minor, Babylon, and Urartu.[62] Although Tabanelli argues that many of the surgical instruments found at Pompeii and Herculaneum are of Etruscan design, he admits their Greek inspiration.[63]

Such evidence as we possess from the Etruscan contribution to early Roman medical ideas is, at best, the subject of reasonable speculation. Like many questions relating to the Etruscans, our evidence can be argued in several lights.[64] One can conclude, reading the religious and legal evidence with care, that the Romans had distinguished between public medical problems, which were handled within the realm of the state religion with its various inherited trappings, and a sort of private medicine, conducted by the *pater familias* as indicated in the tradition recorded by Cato and Pliny.

Other religious aspects of medicine in early Rome resemble those of many early agricultural peoples. There was a goddess, Carna, who protected children against harmful birds during the night.[65] The early Romans recognized special forces as the sources of various diseases. Cicero says that religious attention should not be given to the powers of nature which do harm to man, such as Febris, Tempestates, and Mala Fortuna.[66] There were a great number of divinities who cared for women in childbirth.[67] This kind of outlook is common to the religious-medical origins of many of the Indo-European tribes.[68]

Many later sources, produced in a more sophisticated era, contain traces of early Roman popular medicine. Celsus speaks of various cures which were of a popular nature and were not used by the physician.[69] The strong tradition of Roman popular medicine is illustrated by Celsus' prescription for a toothache, in spite of his assertion of practical experience.[70] Celsus' description of the symptoms of epilepsy is a combination of rational and popular medicine.[71] Scribonius Largus reflects the strength of the traditional medicine by noting, 'this and other treatments of this sort do not have a place in the art of medicine, although they seem helpful to a few.'[72] As with Celsus, Scribonius Largus apparently admits medical solutions which he denies.[73] Serenus Sammonicus castigates these survivals from an earlier era.[74] Such accepted practices must have been widespread in the Republic to be included as a part of general discussion of a later, more educated age. Like Celsus, Serenus mixes his popular and national medicine. He notes that there is a certain sort of fever, which returns on alternate days, 'arranging the attacks with the exactness of an accurate balance', and then he prescribes for it:

> You must seal up in wax the seeds of cummin, minus their tails [and] put this preparation into a bag made of red leather, and put the whole arrangement around the neck of the patient. A branch of pennyroyal, wrapped in wool, will exude healing odours at the time when you expect an attack. Then too, a smashed bug should be eaten with an egg; awful to the touch, it is not difficult to swallow in this fashion.[75]

Other references to popular medicine in the Republic are common, but are repetitious of one another.[76] The Romans had a definite system of medicine before the influx of Greek method and theory, but the native matrix lacked the quality of organization into a generally accepted pattern. The Roman had shown a natural eclecticism in his adaptation of Etruscan practices, and the same characteristic of cultural adaptive genius was to be revealed in regard to Greek ways. The quality of Roman native medicine can be likened, as it evolved, in some aspects to Roman architecture: adaptation with an attempt at cohesion, and a reality of individual purpose.

Agricultural medicine in its simplest setting was modified in many ways soon after Rome became a *polis* and ideas from the Greek world of southern Italy and beyond gradually filtered in through Etruria. Sometimes the contact came directly, although our sources obscure much of the development of anthropomorphic religion among the Etruscans, and archaeology points to a long period of infusion of Greek ideas into Etruria and Rome.[77] After Rome threw out her Etruscan overlords around 500 BC, foreign contacts remained numerous for a short while. Carthage probably recognized Rome as the leading power of central Italy,[78] and the Etruscans lost most of their influence after losing a great naval encounter against the Syracusan Greeks in 474 BC.[79] Greek gods soon arrived to take up residence at Rome, too.

According to Roman traditions, a plague raging in the fifth century BC was stilled by the dedication of a temple to Apollo, and later Apollo *medicus* emerged.[80] Another plague ravaged Rome in

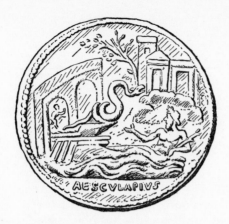

Fig. 1 The reverse of a bronze medallion of Antoninus Pius (AD *138–161*). *Tiber welcomes Asclepius in the form of a snake* (BMC Roman Medallions, *Antoninus Pius, 4*)

295 BC and the Romans decided to recruit the services of the Greek god of medicine. No doubt the Romans had heard of the success of the medical shrines in the Hellenistic world and hoped some of this power might be transferred to Rome.[81] A temple to Asclepius was built on the island in the Tiber, not inside Rome,[82] and this was a reflection of the Roman official suspicion of foreign gods.[83] The pestilence soon went away and the popularity of the new cult was assured.[84] The introduction of Asclepius is the first event of 'medical history' at Rome. Greek physicians quickly followed to serve the rising Roman power, but they form a portion of another segment of the history of Roman medicine.[85]

By the time of the Pyrrhic War, the Romans had a well-defined medical practice on three levels: the private practitioner, recorded by Cassius Hemina,[86] and seen in early Roman law; the 'practical' medicine of the *pater familias* exemplified particularly in the tradition preserved by Cato; and the vague level of Etrusco-Latin religious and magical medicine, which, after the arrival of Asclepius, became amalgamated with Hellenistic religious medical practices.[87]

CHAPTER II

THE BACKGROUND OF
HELLENISTIC MEDICINE

DURING THE FIFTH AND FOURTH centuries BC, the theory and practice of medicine became highly sophisticated in the Greek and Hellenistic world. Greek medicine entered Roman culture after a lengthy development including the observations of the Ionian philosophers, Hippocratic medicine, and Alexandrian anatomy and physiology.[1] Similar to basic development at Rome, Hellenistic medicine had religious and magical, as well as rational, concepts. Among the Greeks, however, the rational approaches were dominant among the educated, whereas Romans of all classes readily used the popular aspects of their native medicine. Despite amazing foresight, the Greeks failed to capitalize upon medicine's potential. As a truly scientific study, it had a short heyday, and non-rational tendencies exerted more influence in the long run than did Hippocratic rationalism.

The Hippocratic *corpus* indicates the Greek genius of synthesis and organization of systems. Medicine was a true 'art', a *techne* which possessed a doctrine developed from rules of practical application into a system. The tendency for ordination is well illustrated by the terse Hippocratic works on the physician's proper deportment and his correct attitude towards his patients. The elaborate advice was expressed in terms understood in the social mood of the day, and the treatises retained archaic phrases as a part of the physician's specialized approaches to his work. The organization of medicine was widespread throughout the Hellenistic world and lurked behind the intellectual backdrop of such as Diocles of Carystus. Specialized physicians appeared as an important segment of Hellenistic life once distinctions were made in the traditional mode of medical treatment, and these differences applied to defined problems within medical practice. The Hippocratic psychological subtlety in the *On the Right Way to Behave* advances several steps with the efforts of Diocles who was 'one of those physicians of subtle and inquiring minds who have something to say about natural science and claim to derive their principles from it'.[2] The study of anatomy had its germs in Diocles' work, but his anatomy was based securely on the observation of animals,[3] as was true for the general considerations of zoological classification from Aristotle. The knowledge of zoology had importance for Diocles in dietetics,[4] and we note specialized work performed on many levels by the descendants of the Hippocratic tradition.

A moot and often discussed question is the social status of the Hellenistic doctor. Plato's well-known reference to slave doctors treating slave patients has recently come under criticism. Plato proves to be unreliable as the final word on the problem, as particularly elucidated by Cohn-Haft and Kudlien.[5] Slave doctors appear to have been the creation of hopeful theories, put forth by Herzog from 'rarely publicized inscriptions . . . which could not be checked'.[6] The medical helper of classical times never was a doctor and did not practise independently even with slave patients. Later the Athenians were expressly to forbid slaves from learning medicine, and Plato's intellectual ideals remain in the realm of the theoretical rather than the actual.[7] None the less, Plato's distinction between the two kinds of medicine puts the modern observer on his guard in regard to the specialization of medical practice as distinguished from the ideal physician who studied philosophy.

There is no doubt surgery became refined in Hellenistic medicine, and was a result of generations of physicians who had accumulated data from their predecessors.[8] Along with gymnasts, dietitians and hygienic experts, they formed the medicine the citizen of the Hellenistic world knew and often respected.[9] The medical men roved about the Hellenistic cities, giving lectures on their topics, and they sought to teach their specialized matter in the sophistic tradition. We receive notices of some of them settling and setting up stalls from which they gave advice and counsel, and these 'offices' were equipped with a supply of sponges and sandals and had provision for running water.[10] We might call this a kind of Hellenistic 'first aid' station, and we can picture the citizens rushing here to have their daily wounds washed and words of reassurance and comfort issued. These were the medical practitioners the public saw in action, but most of them were not educated in the medical specialities characteristic of the Alexandrian Museum. Yet the pattern of medical teaching and research at the Museum had far-reaching influence on how physicians conceived of their work, and the scholarly medicine comparable to philology, poetry, and literature in the Museum determined the specialized techniques of physicians in the Hellenistic world.

Most ordinary persons sought the help of the temple medicine, which had a long tradition in the Greek world. In the Hellenistic world, temples to Asclepius abounded, particularly in Asia Minor. Edelstein's collected testimonia indicate that a vast number of people went to these medical shrines, hoping to be healed by the miraculous intervention of the god.[11] In the same period, spanning the fifth, fourth and third centuries BC, the carefully rational practice of the Hippocratic 'school' of Cos had spread and become more popular as the years went by.[12] By 300 BC, physicians and veterinary surgeons were common, and most cities attempted to procure at least one physician-in-residence, who could be relied upon in his service to the inhabitants.[13] Cities swapped doctors when emergencies arose, and the custom was extended to include circumstances when some of the cities were inundated by throngs attending religious festivals.[14] In such conditions, the health of the general population deteriorated and there was fear that epidemics might occur which could not be controlled.[15] Ample evidence survives attesting the fine service and high ethic of borrowed physicians.[16]

The most honoured of the medical centres was Cos, but there were rational 'schools' of medical instruction long before Cos became renowned. Pergamon, and later Alexandria, asked for Coan physicians to settle and practise, in preference to others with differing training.[17] This is noteworthy as both cities had medical teachers of their own. Once they arrived in their new surroundings, doctors formed clubs like other craft associations. The requirement for membership was medical training at a given centre, such as Cos or Pergamon.[18]

The medical profession, typical of all trained craftsmen in the Hellenistic world, continually moved from place to place, seeking opportunities for employment or more lucrative patrons. Doctors occasionally became politicians to better their lot. Many rulers of the time relied upon physicians' judgement in making decisions.[19] The doctor, as a product of a sophisticated craft whose traditions extended back many generations, found his relationships with the Hellenistic monarchies different from the physician's relation with the *poleis* of Greece. The tiny bit of evidence, for example, available from the Seleucid kingdom suggests a new regard for the doctor by the Hellenistic monarch.[20]

The professional doctor, like his counterparts who specialized in gymnastics and pharmaceuticals, arose from the increasing sophistication of knowledge in the period after Alexander. We find professionals of many kinds, ranging from athletes who competed for a fee to poets who composed on commission. Mercenaries became the usual members of the highly professionalized Hellenistic armies, and the best of the Hellenistic kings surrounded themselves with experts in politics and philosophy. Aristotle's students had forecast the trend as they wrote studies according to classification. Menon's history of medicine as well as Theophrastus' study of plants and drugs suggested that men could no longer master everything as had been the ideal in the classical *polis*. Increasing speciality was well under way among students of medicine by the era of the Hellenistic successor kingdoms. The doctor of the Hippocratic vision no longer sufficed in an age demanding some knowledge of drugs, surgery, dietetics, as well as simple psychology. The enormous expansion of the Greek world after 334 BC made many of the old concepts of education inadequate, and we witness the rise of professional activity with its higher technical achievement but with the breakdown of loyalty to Greek ideals.

Doctors depended upon other crafts in the practice of their art. Archaeological evidence points to increased sophistication of medical implements used in surgery, in conjunction with advances in Hellenistic metallurgy.[21] Physicians relied upon ever-present drug dealers, although most of them could make their own medicaments.[22] Drug fraud was common and there were frequent complaints.[23]

The Ptolemies attempted to control medicine and regulated traffic in worthless drugs. Public medicine was important in Egypt, as distinguished from the medical care in the cities of Asia Minor.[24] The Ptolemies organized medicine as tightly as they had other spheres of social and political life in Egypt.[25] The activities and discoveries of the Museum became common knowledge within the Greek community, and educated men knew some of the philosophical and physical tenets of the Greek doctors in Egypt.[26]

The demands of the Greek settlers made Egypt a combination of the Egyptian past and Greek standards.[27] Most Greeks who came to Egypt lived in Alexandria, or in Ptolemais in the south, and did not settle at will in the *chora*.[28] The great majority of Greek settlers were mercenaries out of a job who were assigned land. In turn they agreed to defend their land and direct its productivity, and they were the Ptolemaic *hoi klerouchoi*. The doctors in the Egyptian *chorai* were supported *ek tou koinou*, that is they were in public or royal service.[29] Traditions for the formal regulation of doctors reached back many centuries in Egypt, and Herodotus tells us Egypt had many physicians in its ancient days.[30] The Ptolemies created a head-tax so the public physicians had adequate means of livelihood.[31]

The first two Ptolemies established the famous Museum in an attempt to make Alexandria the cultural centre of the Hellenistic world. The Ptolemies hoped to enhance their prestige by attracting scholars to Egypt. From the first, the Museum functioned less as a research institution than it did as a showpiece of the Ptolemies' wealth and learning. Ptolemy Philadelphus bought all the books formerly in the collections of Aristotle and Theophrastus, as well as many which he procured from Athens and Rhodes. The Egyptian king wanted to have the largest library in the world, topping even the famous collections of Polycrates of Samos, Peisistratus, the kings of Pergamon, and Euripides.[32] The scholars who flocked to Alexandria found a huge storehouse of scrolls available for their perusal, but it does not follow that they used the library for 'research' in the modern definition. The acquisition of erudition did not produce free questioning nor experimentation,[33] but rather long-winded quarrels among literary pedants who reminded Timon of Philus of 'well-fed bookish birds in a gilded cage'.[34] As Neugebauer has warned, we must beware of turning the Alexandrian Museum into a caricature of a modern post-graduate research institution, with the assumption that the scholars behaved as we expect modern productive scholars to conduct themselves.[35]

The Museum was built into the royal palaces, and had a public walk with exedra provided with seats. Connected to the exedra and their porticos was a large building in which the philosophers and rhetoricians took their common meals. They apparently had some arrangement of holding their property in common, and Ptolemy appointed a 'Priest of the Muses' who directed their work. As a 'Temple of the Muses', the Museum's first loyalty was to poetry and literature, and Alexandrian scholarly production in the first two centuries of the Ptolemaic period mirrored refinement of poetic style and literary collation. The history of the Museum was one of rivalry with Pergamon and her library.[36] Ptolemy Soter had vainly invited Theophrastus and Menander to live in Alexandria, but he managed to gain the poet-scholar Philetas of Cos, and the philosopher Straton, as tutors for his son and eventual successor, Ptolemy Philadelphus. Demetrius of Phaleron may have instilled the idea to found a library in Alexandria as an attraction to poets and scholars of all sorts, and Ptolemy Philadelphus continued his father's designs with further emphasis on his own half-learning in zoology.[37] Although we must substitute reasonable speculation for solid evidence, it seems Philadelphus' dilettantism in zoology led to the encouragement of such as Herophilus and Erasistratus.

The important labour at the Museum consisted in establishing correct and reliable texts of the major Greek authors. Hippocrates

was among those considered, and a certain Mnemon of Side
(Pamphylia) brought a rare manuscript of the Hippocratic 'school'
for the collection in the library.[38] Ptolemy Euergetes obtained the
official texts of the three great Athenian tragedians through deception, as related in a delightful anecdote by Galen.[39] Erudition and
criticism, rather than spontaneous creativity, comprised the
general activity within the Museum, and the first participants in
the Museum were poet-scholars or philosopher-scientists with
only some attempt at specialized knowledge. Theocritus' friend
Nicias was a doctor who wrote reasonably elegant epigrams, some
of which survive in the *Greek Anthology*. In one, Nicias writes
with poignancy of the fear women had at childbirth.[40] Theocritus may have had some medical knowledge as certain words he
uses appear to have traces of medical terminology.[41] Nicias
receives the dedication of Theocritus' Idylls XI, XIII, and
XXVIII, and the last two refer to him as living in Miletus. Nicias
probably frequented the medical teaching areas at Cos,[42] but
there is no basis for connecting Theocritus' father Praxagoras with
the famous physician of that name.

Later scholars appeared at Alexandria who made no pretence of
being poets, although the tendency had set in for doctors to pursue
poetry as well.[43] Doctors wrote critical studies of Hippocrates,
books on the art of cookery, investigations of traditional superstition, perfumes, proper arrangement of wreaths, banquets, as
well as drugs and diet, and the approaches of medical practice.[44]
Diocles and Diphilus of Siphnos had become famous for their
works on many subjects before the creation of the Alexandrian
Museum,[45] and the physicians at Alexandria continued in their
paths. Of course Diocles, Diphilus and Praxagoras wrote much on
medicine, but it appeared in the context of 'investigation' or
'philosophy' rather than completely segregated into a category of
'physicians' services'.[46] These physicians remembered Hippocrates' maxim on the limits of their art,[47] yet attempted to integ-
rate as much knowledge as possible into the scope of their investigation. None the less, their 'research' tended to be bookish rather
than experimental, and the tradition of Hellenistic medicine—
with the important but unusual exceptions of Herophilus and

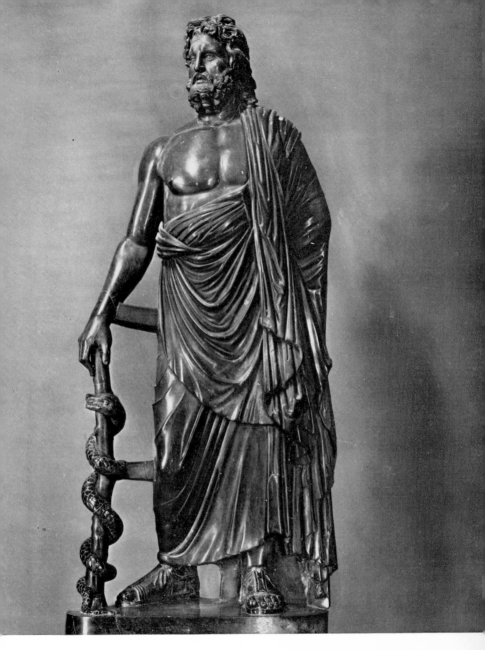

1 Life-size bronze statue of Aesculapius found at Antium (modern Anzio), mid-second century AD. The staff with its encircling snake is the expected symbol associated with the cult all over the Roman world. Probably a Roman copy of a Hellenistic original. Capitoline Museum, Rome.

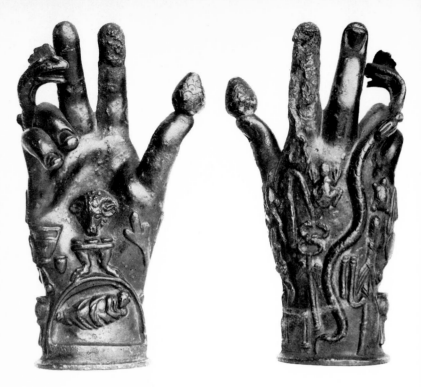

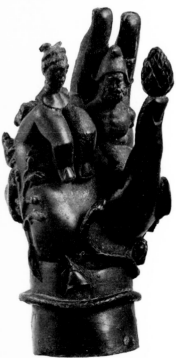

2–4 Roman bronze hands whose symbols appear to have magico-religious and medical significance. Among the mixture one observes connections with Mithras (the pine cone), the Dioscuri (a cap with star), Hermes and his symbol (head with winged headdress and winged caduceus). The snake has obvious medical connections and possibly the frog, turtle and beetle suggest efficacious potion ingredients. British Museum and Avenches Museums.

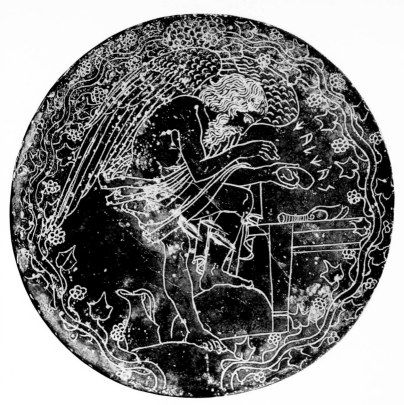

5, 6 Two examples in bronze of the Etruscan practice of haruspication, or reading livers for omens. The bronze mirror back shows a winged seer examining a liver, freshly cut from the carcass of a sacrificed animal. Fourth century BC. The bronze liver from Piacenza probably shows, in the style of a map, the liver with its parts as they would be associated with various regions of the sky. Each section in relation to the sky would indicate favourable or unfavourable omens. It is suggested that this is based on earlier Babylonian practice. Vatican and Piacenza Museums.

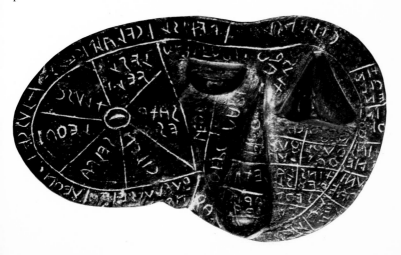

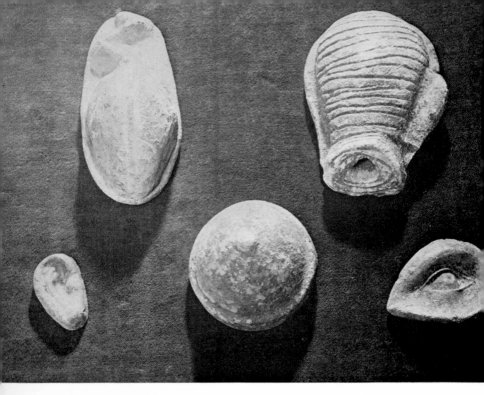

7 Etruscan terracotta votives from the temple of Veii. Included here are what appear to be a uterus, a breast and a right ear. Kansas University Medical Center.

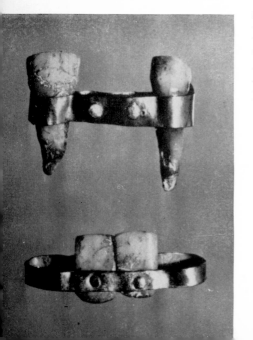

8 Examples of Etruscan dental practice. The technique seems to be to fashion a primitive bridge using a gold band to span the gap between the live teeth. To this band would then be riveted the patient's 'dead teeth' with their roots sawn off. City of Liverpool Museums.

9, 10 Medical or erotic themes as illustrated on an Etruscan bucchero vase. It has been suggested that the drawings may not be contemporary with the vase. *Right*, the physician (?) appears to be about to begin a gynecological examination; *below*, the patient is about to receive an enema from the physician (?) who administers it with a tube attached to a vessel which he holds aloft in his left hand.

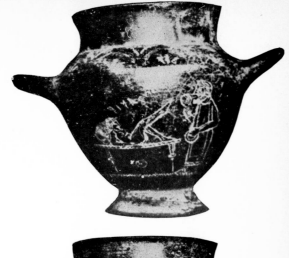

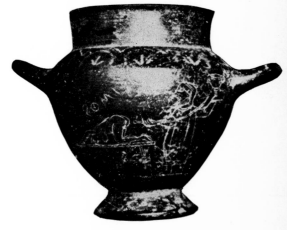

11 *Discus* of a Roman terracotta lamp, probably of Italian origin, early first century AD. The scene represented may be from a lost, erotic comedy which probably satirized the pompous physician who paraded his fine tools without actually knowing their use. The pincers which the bald-headed physician (Hippocrates or Socrates caricatured?) applies are of a type seen in Plate 35. The operation being performed may be a farcical view of the Jewish custom of circumcision. Similar examples are known from Tarsus and in the Benacchi collection, Athens. British Museum.

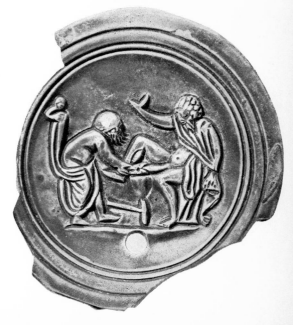

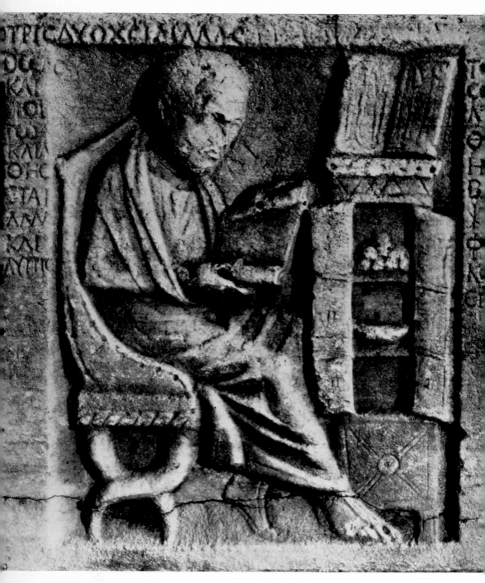

12 Late Hellenistic relief from Ostia illustrating the Roman philosopher-physician sitting in his study. He reads a scroll, taken from the cabinet on the right, which holds others and a bowl. On top of it is a stylized representation of his open instrument case with the instruments inside (*cf*. Plate 14). Ostia Museum.

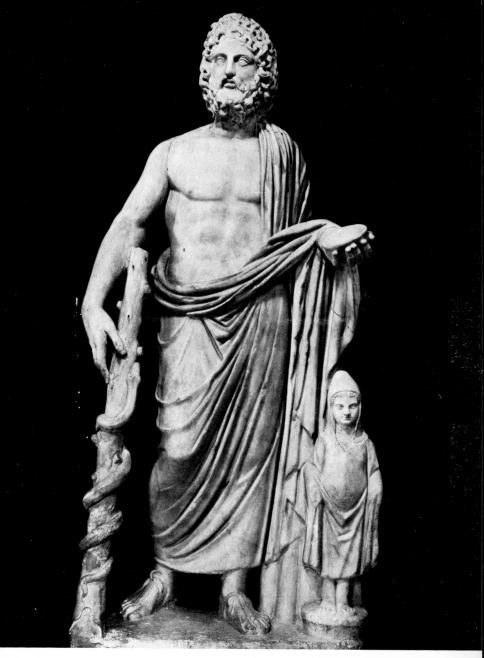

13 Marble statue of Aesculapius holding his staff with snake and a patera in his left hand. The small Telesphorus figure beside him shows clearly the association within the cult of Life, Death and Sleep. The 'temple-sleep', or incubation, was a feature of the cult throughout the Roman Empire (*see* Fig. 11). Second century AD. Borghese Museum, Rome.

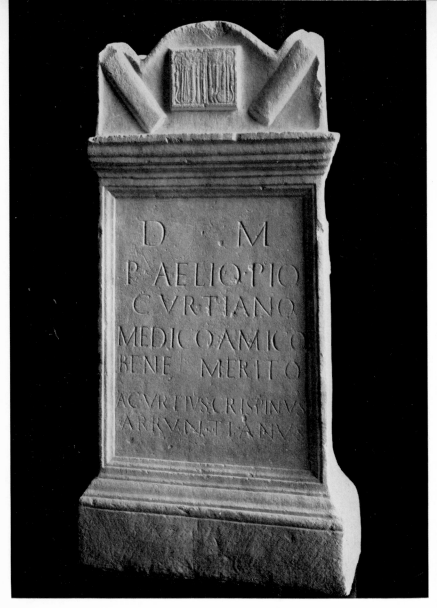

14 Roman marble funerary stele of the second century AD dedicated to Publius Aelius Pius Curtianus. He was apparently the freedman or slave doctor of Curtius Crispinus Arruntianus. At the top is seen an open instrument case with the instruments faithfully represented. On either side are probably stylized representations of the same case closed.

Erasistratus—formed around a series of physicians' commentaries upon earlier works.

The bookish doctor became a stock character in popular satire long before Martial, Lucian, and Plutarch.[48] Panaretus, a philosopher who lived at the court of Ptolemy Euergetes and received twelve talents a year for his presence, was happy to boast he never needed a doctor for any reason.[49] Nor was the physician particularly respected at the Alexandrian court. A certain Chrysippus, son of Chrysippus the teacher of Erasistratus, was remembered because he had been flogged by Ptolemy on a false charge, and humiliated by being dragged around the court like a common criminal.[50] The doctors and other scholars did not always enjoy the good will of their patrons, and probably endured much interference in their work, which was directed by Ptolemy through his appointed Priest of the Muses. Plutarch records the meddling of the infamous Ptolemy Euergetes II (Physcon).[51] 'Ptolemy masqueraded as a lover of learning and [his scholars] quibbled with him about an insignificant verse, or about a word, or an historical instance far into the night. But when Ptolemy was excessively cruel or violent . . . none of his scholars offered objection.'[52]

The popular accounts of the famous names and wonder-tales about the medical faculty at Alexandria are generally unreliable.[53] Two names, however, stand out as important and unusual in medical studies. The first of the two, Herophilus of Chalcedon, worked in the Museum under Ptolemy Soter and possibly in the first years of the reign of Ptolemy Philadelphus.[54] Herophilus was of the Coan tradition and followed the work of Praxagoras. Galen considers Herophilus a clear thinker, using a kind of logical method as contrasted to 'empiricism', and this led to what Galen calls 'obscurity' in the interpretation of Herophilus' work by later physicians.[55] Galen usually praises Herophilus for the care of his work and his combination of shrewd observation and sound reasoning.[56]

The relation of gymnastics to the study of anatomy formed an important section of Herophilus' concepts of general anatomy. If we can trust the tradition preserved in Galen, Herophilus attempted to apply a careful study of exercises to remedies for a

c

given disease, as well as to infuse his study of anatomy with the application of diet for good health.[57] But it was to the study of anatomy that Herophilus was mainly devoted, and his efforts were good enough to earn the commendation from Galen that 'nobody did more in this until the time of Marinus and Numesianus'.[58] Herophilus' work was well in line with the desire of the Ptolemies for 'practical discoveries' at the Museum,[59] and his tract *On Dietetics* was an important practical treatise.[60] It dealt at length with his opinions of drugs, diet, and hygiene.

Human cadavers were dissected at Alexandria,[61] and Herophilus made important discoveries, such as the demonstration of the origin and course of nerves from the brain and spinal column.[62] Following the Coan-Praxagorean pattern, Herophilus thought the brain was the seat of sensation, and he put the central point in the ventricles of the brain.[63] This was a conclusion from his belief that the brain was the centre of the nervous system.[64] Herophilus' acceptance of the four Hippocratic humours showed in his classifications of the four major functions of the body. There was nourishment, or the nourishing soul, which had its origins in the liver. Secondly, there was heat and animal power, or the warming soul which resided in the heart. The third category, the thinking soul, had its seat in the brain. Sensation and motion originated in the nerves.[65] Herophilus described the eye, which he carefully dissected,[66] and made the use of the pulse in diagnosis understandable.[67]

Herophilus had a long-lasting influence, as Galen indicates. Galen depended upon Herophilus for numerous anatomical and philosophical conclusions, brought forth during the short period of brilliance in medical research at Alexandria. It was this era which advanced medicine in the Greek mould well enough to hold its place in the Roman Empire.[68]

Erasistratus, the second of the two better-known Alexandrian medical researchers, provides another view of the brilliant tradition, and the philosophical problems of Hellenistic medicine as it came to the Romans. Commonly called 'The Father of Physiology', Erasistratus came after Herophilus, in medical research at the Alexandrian Museum.[69] He received some training in the 'schools' of 'atomic theory', as well as instruction from the Cnidian 'school' concerning physiology and the pneuma.[70] Erasistratus contested Aristotle's theories relating to the heart being the seat of man's intelligence, and he discovered and demonstrated that the tendinous elongations of the dura mater had some sort of pith in them.[71] He traced them to their origins in the brain.[72] Fascinating was his work on the problems of the circulation, and Erasistratus came close to making monumental discoveries, which waited until the seventeenth century and Harvey to be expounded fully.[73] Erasistratus felt there was a kind of lifegiving substance (*pneuma*) in the blood, and following his teachers, Praxagoras and Chrysippus, he saw little else in the arterial circulation.[74] Erasistratus demonstrated the function of the epiglottis, seen by Aristotle, but the Alexandrian demolished the notion accepted to his day concerning the epiglottis and its role in providing food for the pneuma. Plato had thought some food and liquid passed into the lungs so there would be something to give nourishment to the pneuma.[75] Erasistratus supposed all tissue had a triple function, and proved to his own satisfaction that the artery's purpose was to carry pneuma.[76] The vein had the function of carrying food, and the nerve was for the pneuma of sensation.[77] He was a rare anatomical expert in the medicine of the Hellenistic world, and our sources indicate that he carried his work to the point of vivisection, or the application of a remedy directly to an organ exposed in the body of a patient.[78]

The practice of medicine in the Hellenistic world was well developed, and it had evolved in several differing patterns. Democritus helped to formulate theories absorbed by the Coan 'school', and eventually gave rise to the theories of the pneuma, seen especially in the remnants of Praxagoras' writings. There was the school of thought, following the Academy at Athens and Aristotle, which assumed that man's intelligence had its seat in the heart, and other functions were located elsewhere. The heritage of earlier Egyptian embalming practices was involved in the background of Ptolemaic encouragement for anatomical investigation. Nevertheless, the restless Greek spirit of inquiry and theorizing was the base of the phenomenon we see in Alexandrian medicine and anatomy.

For some yet unexplained reason, the direct examination of the human body was curtailed after about two or three generations of momentous progress. Probably religious prohibition was involved, and it may be in the spirit of general disgust that Celsus and Caelius Aurelianus tell their brutal tales of vivisection at Alexandria.

Tradition recorded the name of Ptolemy Physcon (or 'Kakergetes') as the author, in the second century BC, of the great dispersion of Alexandrian philosopher-scientists throughout the Mediterranean world. He murdered some of them, but sent most of them into exile. They included grammarians, philosophers, mathematicians, musicians, painters, athletic trainers, physicians, and many others 'of skill in their profession'.[79] They were forced by poverty to teach what they knew and no longer were able to depend on stipends from the Ptolemaic court.

Tracing the course of late Hellenistic medical thought is difficult if not impossible. Wellmann devotes much effort in an attempt to determine just when the famous Heracleides of Tarentum did practise, and from whom he received his basic inspiration and instruction.[80] Galen indicates his open admiration for Heracleides,[81] because he had clarified the Alexandrian physicians' work on the pulse. Names such as Zenon, Mantias, Serapion, Philotimus, Evenor, Nileus, Molpis, Nymphodorus, Andreas, and Protarchus appear in the traditional network between Alexandria and the late Roman Republic, but their exact chronological relationship remains vexed.[82] The body-physician of Antiochus III, to cite one example, receives recognition for his recipes and was an 'Erasistratean'.[83]

In many areas of the ancient classical world, Greek medicine and its corresponding philosophical, religious, and rational legacy had an extraordinary attractiveness to native cultures. Like so many of the gifts the Greeks gave to the Mediterranean world, Greek and Hellenistic medicine became modified and transmuted by the tempering resident culture. Examples are numerous of the widespread activity of cultural transfer. Egypt has been noted. Sicily and southern Italy evolved an independent tradition of medicine, Greek in spirit and direction, but having qualities suggesting native drive.[84] The area between Asia Minor and India altered medical ideas under the impact of the Greek cultural veneer and recast them into new forms.[85] Distant as it was, India felt Greek influence, and Indian culture, much as the Roman, was changed in ways that were sometimes imperceptible, yet profound.[86] As in Rome in many respects, so too in India native abilities emerged as dominant in the cultural tussle.

Rome was one of the many fringe areas affected by the Hellenistic cultural explosion, but unlike India she was to inherit far more Hellenization, particularly after Rome incorporated Greece into her empire. In the late Republic and early Empire, the resultant 'Greco-Roman' pattern of life was a fusion rather than a conquest. Greco-Roman medicine was a product of long years of Hellenistic theory and practice joined with strong native Roman medical experience. After the arrival of Greek physicians in Rome, the Roman bent directed Greek traditions into new moulds. In supplying a practical drive to medicine, the Romans made contributions of their own in the application of hygiene and sound medicine on a wide scale. Hellenistic medical thought gave a cohesion which native Roman medicine lacked, but which the Roman rapidly adapted to fit his own needs.

CHAPTER III

HELLENISTIC MEDICINE IN THE ROMAN WORLD

IN THE COURSE OF ITS RISE to power in the west, the Roman Republic attracted many Greek doctors. In 219 BC, Archagathus came to Rome from the Peloponnesus, and from this time Greek 'rational' and theoretical medicine influenced Roman approaches. Earlier Greek medical ideas may have crept into Rome from Sicily and southern Italy, but evidence for this matter is slight.[1] Early in the third century BC, the Romans adopted Asclepius as one of their gods, and Rome came to know much of Hellenistic religious medicine so closely aligned with the common practice of medicine.

Before turning to the formal 'schools' of Greek medicine practised among the Romans, we might well look at an extraordinary individual whose success in adapting Greek medical principles to a Roman audience throws light on the desires of that audience. This was Asclepiades, who came to Rome about a century after Archagathus with the intention of making his mark as a rhetorician. His career in rhetoric was apparently short and he saw greater opportunities in medicine. Soon he established himself as a respected physician whose practice among the Romans differed markedly from that of Archagathus. Asclepiades' link with Erasistratus was Cleophantus, a surgeon and gynaecologist of distinction, and Cleophantus provided the rhetorician-turned-physician with inspiration and points of reference in his writings.[2]

Pliny gives us solid indications why Asclepiades succeeded in his new profession, at least as the Roman viewed it in the context of Hellenistic cultural influence. Asclepiades' good sense and practical approaches made more difference to the Roman than most of the Hellenistic medical theory. The Greeks originally made use of sound medical principles, but when Hellenistic physicians arrived in Rome, 'experience—that most effective teacher of all subjects, particularly medicine—had degenerated into words and babbling.'[3] Pliny further sneers at those who 'found it pleasant to sit listening to lectures [on medicine]', and at the sort of medicine which 'survived to claim only a part of its former sphere'.[4]

At first glance, the image of Asclepiades as the successful self-taught physician appears to contrast sharply with the Greek medical sources who quote heavily from Asclepiades' works.[5] A closer look, however, at references from Galen, Soranus, and others, reveals copious quotation, usually to refute Asclepiades. Galen caps most statements on Asclepiades when he writes, '[Asclepiades] tries to contradict [Hippocrates] in something he knows absolutely nothing about, and, I might add, in moronic, idiotic language.'[6] Pliny is unhappy about Asclepiades' unscrupulous methods, and the Hellenistic physicians condemn him for lack of theoretical medicine. Yet Pliny gives the over-all impression Asclepiades did what he could with 'a brilliant mind able to cope with matters other than rhetoric', and so Asclepiades 'switched from rhetoric to medicine'. Asclepiades recognized five principles of general application in his system of medicine, which was 'reduced to the discovery of causes and a process of guess-work'.[7]

Asclepiades is particularly fascinating as he represents the medical application of the theories of Democritus and Epicurus. When the later Roman philosopher-physicians quote from the works of Asclepiades, they do so with great agitation in order to prove that his mechanistic system was incorrect. The atomistic theories, presented in Latin by Lucretius, were in vogue when Asclepiades 'discovered' medicine. Much as Galen was to complain later about Asclepiades,[8] Lucretius' observations were visual rather than logical. The kind of medicine which emerged from such conclusions infuriated Galen and sometimes puzzled, sometimes disturbed Pliny.[9] Pliny, rather than Galen and the Hellenistic philosopher-physicians, realizes the real importance of the practice of Asclepiades in Rome, although Pliny attempts to disguise it. 'Above all else [Asclepiades] was aided by the magical nonsense which was widespread enough to negate [the Roman] faith in his traditional medicine [i.e. the use of herbs],' and '[Asclepiades] had great success because of the very crude and disgusting cures of ancient medicine.' Of course Pliny accuses Asclepiades of 'inventing nonsense even beyond the Magi', but he attracted many patients by the elimination of harsh treatment in many diseases, and by his eloquent and much-practised oratory. Democritus figures in the discussion, which shows Pliny's recognition of the atomistic philosophy behind Asclepiades. The attraction to Romans of this method is clearly indicated, as Asclepiades provided a system 'that everyone thought he could provide for himself, and everyone cheered him as having revealed that the most easily understood matters were also the truth.' Simple remedies were the hallmark of Asclepiades, who is called by Pliny (quoting Varro), the 'cold-water giver', and by the *Anonymus Londinensis*, the 'wine giver'. He won a great repute by applying broad remedies to a number of diseases, or as Pliny suggests, 'to relieve sickness or to bring on sleep'.[10]

Asclepiades followed some of the precepts of Erasistratus and Cleophantus, and he disregarded any sort of strenuous remedies. He conformed to nature's dictates as far as he saw them, and analysed each patient in light of his experience.[11] He was a master of image-building, and his popularity was great among his Roman patients, who found him willing to listen and learn. The Romans remembered him in striking contrast to Archagathus.[12]

Asclepiades advocated physical treatments, as sweating baths in dropsy, and he used what he thought best from the medical writings of the Greek and Hellenistic world.[13] His treatment for dropsy was taught by Chrysippus the Cnidian, and Asclepiades questioned the authority of the physiologist Erasistratus, and even Hippocrates.[14] A kindly rationalism was one of his major qualities.

Asclepiades in his book *On Dropsy* holds that in cases where fluid has already gathered, whether in small or large amount, but has not yet spread to the feet or the legs, an athlete's regimen should be prescribed, with considerable walking and running. . . . But if the fluid spreads to the lower parts, he forbids much exercise and also the use of purgatives and diuretics.[15]

Asclepiades prescribes wine for those suffering with fever, with the exercise of discretion. . . . He holds that the appropriate time for treatment is more likely to be created by the skilful physician than to appear by itself or by the will of the gods. . . . In his *Rules of Health* he recommends variation of the mode of the life . . . he holds that there is no digestion of food in our bellies but that the food is broken down in the belly undigested and passes through the several parts of the body, evidently penetrating all the fine passages . . . the soul, he says, is no thing but the combination of all the senses . . . he declares there is nothing without a cause.[16]

Celsus notes how Asclepiades changed Roman opinions of Greek doctors. As a Roman, his remarks are revealing.

But after those mentioned above, no one troubled themselves concerning anything at all other than to examine what had gone before until Asclepiades altered in great measure the consideration of healing.[17]

Asclepiades practised a clinical medicine appealing to the Romans, because he chose to deal directly with his patients rather than expounding medical theory. Asclepiades was influenced by his Roman environment, and he was Roman in practical application of medicine. His synthetic methods are strikingly similar to those of Celsus. Celsus, speaking as a lay physician in the tradition of the *Pater familias*, says, 'It is through these men especially that our beneficial profession has matured.'[18]

Asclepiades represents the process of adaptation and he stands in the gap between the Hellenistic theoretical approaches and Latin practical medicine. If Asclepiades was a rhetorician by training, his success in medicine indicates the basic nature of Roman medicine, and the manner the Romans thought of it. Asclepiades leads directly into Celsus' encyclopedia, which is a product of a layman, but a layman who educated himself in the best medicine of his day, and could take his place with the best of practising physicians in Rome. Asclepiades' unmedical background, similar to Celsus', allowed the utilization of the best that a sharp mind could see in medical theory. The Greeks, with their not dissimilar rational patterns, provided a method of direction of the Latin practical drive and, after Asclepiades, the Roman practice and adaptation of the Greek theories became customary.

The Greek medical theories, adapted by Asclepiades, were but a part of a vast mélange of Greek and Hellenistic philosophical concepts which gave birth to a number of sophisticated views of man. A basic change from the earlier, narrowly conceived Greek conceptualization was characteristic in medical speculation from Hippocrates onward.[19] A pervasive Stoicism prepared the Greek world for Empire, well in advance of the Romans.[20] In the west, Latin culture was dominant, and its mould determined social, political, and intellectual life. The Latin tradition produced skilled synthesizers of Hellenistic patterns, and the writings of Cicero and Celsus, and the practice of Asclepiades indicated successful fusion of Hellenistic philosophies with Latin methods and framework of reference. By the reign of Trajan, the Roman practical drive destroyed differences between medical theories, and the Roman found the best medicine was in adaptation of Hellenistic precepts. This is noteworthy in Roman practices of contraception which may have had far-reaching results.

In general, the Roman mistrusted the Hellenistic physician with his fancy theories. The Latin practical ability failed to perceive the value of theoretical speculation, and, by and large, left theory in the hands of the Greek physicians. On the other hand, the Romans had great respect for the theories forming part of the Hellenistic cultural heritage. The masters of the Early Empire absorbed as much of the Greek ways as was practical, but we are left with a general impression that the Roman accepted Hellenistic ideals as an outward veneer, and retained the Latin practical base for solving his problems. Thus, what appears at first glance to be wholehearted Roman acceptance of Greek ideas is revealed, on closer inspection, to be careful Roman separation of the cultural from the practical.

Turning to the Hellenistic theories of medicine, we note the general Roman enthusiasm for Greek culture, and Diocles of Carystos was associated with Aristotle, and Praxagoras of Cos was viewed with as much respect as the great names in Greek philosophy and literature.[21] The Roman ignored the importance of philosophical as well as medical training for the Greek doctor.[22] The intellectual traditions of the Hellenistic east continued in their independent paths, much as the political ones did within the matrix of the imperial settlement. The medical centres at Cos and Alexandria flourished, but were feeble reflections of the great days of the Hellenistic kingdoms.

In the Hellenistic 'schools' themselves, the followers of the two famous Alexandrian physicians, Herophilus and Erasistratus, found it was easier to theorize about medicine as a philosophy than to imitate the methods of their meticulous forerunners.[23] There were exceptions, of course. Newly founded medical centres operated for a time, after the peak of Hellenistic prosperity, as those under Zeuxis at Laodicaea and Hicesius at Smyrna.[24] By Cicero's day, differences between the Herophileans and the followers of Erasistratus had disappeared. After this point, those who espoused Herophilus distinguished themselves by asserting that the Hippocratic writings were the all-time authority in medical practice; the opposing 'school' spoke harshly of Hippocrates.

As the complex heritage of the Hellenistic medical world emerged into the early Roman Empire, the compendia of generations of the medico-philosophical arguments came to be labelled 'schools'.[25] By the end of the first century BC, the medical sect known as the 'Dogmatists' had become important. In general terms, the Dogmatists emphasized the study of anatomy, and defended their position by reference to Platonic, Aristotelian, Stoic, and Epicurean systems. A second 'school', the Empiricists, flatly rejected the idea that the physician could detect the unknown functional origins of the body, or that such knowledge would be beneficial for medical practice. They placed full reliance upon philosophical argument, and were known in their own time as the medical *skeptikoi*, who offered opinions.[26]

An interpretation of the Hippocratic writings gave birth to a third 'school'. Throughout the Hippocratic treatise *On Ancient Medicine* is the assertion that man's nature, in the main, consists of his own individuality. Calling themselves Methodists, physicians of the late Hellenistic and early Roman Imperial periods, who argued from this point of view, rejected all generalities in medicine. In the Methodistic concept, the physician insisted that the primary objective of medicine was the individual patient, and phenomena as they were observed in the individual were the only realities of medicine. This sect was associated with the revived philosophy of Pyrrho, and it rejected all general knowledge, saying it was led only by the Present. The view partially counteracted the Hellenistic presumption for the typical and normal neglect of the particular.[27] Themison, as a disciple of Asclepiades, systematized his master's writings, and is usually given credit for 'founding' the Methodist sect.[28] As a philosophy of medicine, it became important among Greek physicians in the Roman Empire. Among adherents to this 'school' were the charlatan Thessalus of Tralles, the great gynaecologist Soranus of Ephesus, and the compiler Caelius Aurelianus.[29]

A fourth 'school' arose from a variation within the Dogmatic teachings, in the form of the Pneumatists, who harked back to the principles of the *pneuma*, as taught by Aristotle and Erasistratus.[30] The Pneumatic concept, probably formulated by Athenaeus of Attalia, had the precepts of Stoicism interwoven into its assertions. Similar to the Stoics, they rejected materialism and taught that there was a primordial matter, the *pneuma*, from which all life came. They revived the Hippocratic notion of the four humours, and said a disturbance in the humours was a disturbance in the proper balance of the *pneuma* in the human body, and thus was the cause of disease.[31]

In the course of development of the medical and philosophical theories in the early Roman Empire, the Roman overlay became more apparent. Although the practice of medicine in the early Empire never attained the status of a universally accepted progressive 'science', it did evolve into some semblance of outward unity among those who became 'eclectics'.[32] The Roman practical drive altered the traditional form of philosophical medical concepts, forcing a kind of unity upon similar medical theories. Even the Methodistic training of Soranus, and the consequent popularity of his approach in the Latin west, indicated a superficial unity with a latent dichotomy between east and west.

'Eclecticism' was the usual pattern that emerged in the practice of formal medicine in the Roman Empire after AD 100. Wellmann stops his account of the Pneumatic school with the appearance of Archigenes of Apamea, and Galen notes how Archigenes combined many approaches.[33] Although Antonius Musa and Agathinus of Sparta exhibited the Eclectic outlook, Eclecticism was not delineated until Archigenes. The sceptical tone, characteristic of Celsus, appears in the writings of Aretaeus of Cappadocia, who borrows much from Archigenes.[34] Roman common sense overcame the Hellenistic predilection for medical theory.[35]

The Greek compendium, however, left its mark on Roman medicine. The sorry examples cited by Stahl were the results of worshipping the antiquarian past which marred scholarly efforts in the Roman Empire. In these terms, Galen shaped the medical world after his day into dogmatic and Roman Eclectic patterns, and his preponderant influence cast Roman medicine after AD 200. Soranus' influence remained strong in the west, but in epitome, and it is this leftover medicine Stahl criticizes.[36] In practice, it was difficult to tell one sect from the other by the reign of Trajan.

The four 'schools' (Methodist, Empiric, Dogmatic, Pneumatic) which merged into an unconscious fusion in the second century, and which Galen exemplified in its final Eclectic form, had common elements. In the writings of Herodotus, the combination of many factors in medical theory shows clearly.[37] Herodotus was of Methodist training and background, but the remains of his writing reflect the continuing process of amalgamation. The Roman imperial world provides its stamp. Herodotus showed his Greek background by incorporation of Hellenistic theoretical concepts, but the tone of his work is of the Roman Empire and of Roman practicality.

> If one is to investigate the blood, one must procure it from the patient from the crook of the arm, and the syringe be filled in

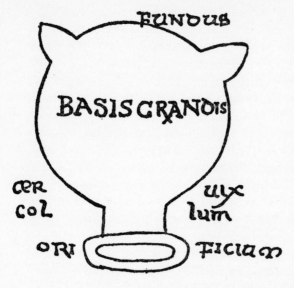

FUNDUS

BASIS GRANDIS

CER COL

ULX LUM

ORI FICIUM

Fig. 2 Illustration of the uterus from the Latin summary of Soranus by Muscio (MS. c. AD 850). It is a good example of the survival of anatomical concepts borrowed by Galen and Soranus from the Alexandrian tradition. The famous 'horns' do not appear (cf. Galen, VIII, 889) in the diagram, although their existence was accepted (on Galen's authority until the naissance. Vide Fig. 14, p. 129; Galen, II, 890; Soranus, I, 57 (after Singer)

correct measure, as it is suitable for the patient. The incision may act as a sacrificial cleansing of everything harmful for the patient. But if he should become unconscious, and be hot to the touch, then one should use the cupping-glass for slow bleeding, and apply soothing lotions, plasters and relaxants . . . one should then get the patient to drink some fresh wine to counteract the heated jaundice of the liver.[38]

Unfortunately, Herodotus' work, and others like it, were easily adapted into a rule-book which probably gave some Roman readers the false notion they were qualified physicians after they had read them.[39]

The Methodist 'school's' finest example was Soranus of Ephesus, and his *Gynecology* continued in the mood of Celsus and Hippocrates. Soranus, although he proclaimed his Methodist training and outlook, also revealed the Roman Empire in which he lived. The handbook custom had become commonplace by his day, and he wrote his *Gynecology* as a guidebook for midwives.[40] Probably Soranus was addressing female 'physicians', that is those who dealt solely with female diseases.[41]

The care of pregnant women has three stages . . . when conception has taken place, one must beware of every excess and change both bodily and psychic. For the seed is evacuated through fright, sorrow, sudden joy and generally by severe mental upset; through vigorous exercise . . . by the administration of drugs . . . through want, indigestion, drunkenness, vomiting, diarrhoea . . .[42]

A suitable [midwife] will be literate, with her wits about her, possessed of a good memory, loving work, respectable and generally not unduly handicapped as regards her senses, sound of limb, robust, and according to some people, endowed with long slim fingers and short nails at her fingertips. She must be literate in order to comprehend the art through theory, too. . . .[43]

In spite of the impact of the Roman milieu, the theoretical base was still important for the physician trained in the Hellenistic mould. Although Roman practical motives dominate Soranus' work, he maintains his cloak of Hellenism, and, to some extent, forces his medicine into preconceived theoretical form. This tendency baffled Roman patients, and caused them to seek other solutions.

Rufus of Ephesus, as a representative of the Pneumatic 'school', exhibited a medical method both synthetic and eclectic. His medicine showed the problems noted with Soranus: a fine objective spirit with a necessary forcing of medical practice into the Greek philosophical straitjacket. Rufus' treatise, *On Interrogation of the Patient*, indicates his awareness of the problems the Hellenistic method raised. He pleads for breadth of vision in medicine which the philosophical base sometimes prevented.

One must put questions to the patient, for thereby certain aspects of the disease can be better understood, and the treatment rendered more effective. And I place the interrogation of the patient himself first, since in this way you can learn how far his mind is healthy or otherwise; and you can get some idea of the disease and the part affected. . . . This is a very important diagnostic point.[44]

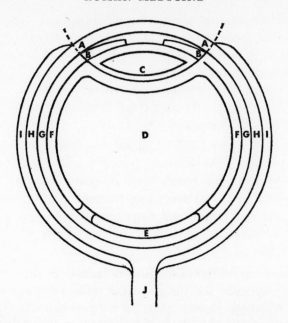

Fig. 3 Diagram of the structures of the eye based on Rufus of Ephesus, c. AD 150 (see Rufus, pp. 136, 154, 170, 464 (from Rhazes)). A cornea; B iris; C lens; D vitreous humour; E retina; F arachnoid layer; G choroid layer; H sclerotic layer; I conjunctiva; J optic nerve. This surprisingly accurate description was ignored in the medieval transmission as seen in Vesalius' diagram of the eye

I admire Hippocrates for his ingenious method; undoubtedly a great many fine discoveries have been made by it. At the same time, I advise anyone wishing for an exact knowledge in these various matters not to neglect the method of interrogation.[45]

Rufus continually reveals his roots in Greek philosophical speculation. The humours figure heavily in diagnosis and treatment.[46] Rufus used for diagnosis what modern man calls 'moods'. These basic categories, such as the 'black mood'[47] which would result from the overabundance of black bile in the body, were given prime importance in medical theory among the Hellenistic sects in the Roman Empire.[48]

Galen, the most prolific of all the physicians in antiquity, states often the problems he has in conveying what he is doing to his public. He derides the factionalism that divides medicine, and it is 'a most oppressive problem to eliminate, and it resists all efforts to clean it up, and is much harder to cure than an itch'.[49] He notes the real danger within the Hellenistic approach, and yet uses the opportunity to present his own view. 'Those [physicians] who are slaves to their sects not only have no firm knowledge of health, but, in addition, they will not stop to learn,' and '[they] ignore the skill of nature and refuse to learn.'[50]

Galen should be regarded as an over-all summary of medical practice and theory, within Hellenistic concepts. He is the great consolidation of Greco-Roman medicine, and put into his volumes about everything that was worth preserving of the theory and practice of medicine which had emerged from Greece and had undergone various changes to the second century. As with Aretaeus and Rufus, Galen's medicine is learned in philosophical jargon and sometimes based upon shrewd observation. Galen attempted to verify by dissection some of the anatomical theories handed down to him, apparently with various animals. Possibly, however, Galen possessed greater knowledge of human anatomy than he wished to be openly known.[51]

Singer rightly observes, 'the very bulk of Galen's writings cuts us off from adequate historical judgement of his predecessors.'[52] But we can gain a rather clear picture of Galen's concept of medical practice, as it is sandwiched into the various tracts on drugs, anatomy, and what we would label physiology.[53] Book II of the *On Anatomical Procedures* shows the eclecticism of Galen as well as the heritage in which he operated.

> I commend Marinus, who has written on anatomical pro-
> cedure, without criticizing my other predecessors who did
> not. For them it was superfluous to compose memoranda for
> themselves or for others since they practised dissection from
> childhood under parental instruction, as they did reading and
> writing. And it was not only professional physicians among
> our predecessors who studied anatomy, but also general
> philosophers.[54]

D

This is the ideal presented by Galen, and the picture of 'children studying anatomy' is pure fiction, supposedly borrowed from legends of the 'Asclepiadae' then current at Pergamon.[55] Philosophers who studied anatomy came from a long-standing tradition that such as Democritus and others in pre-Socratic times had studied medicine.[56] Galen makes clear what the state of medicine was like in his own day.

> . . . the art came to be customarily imparted not only to kinsmen but to those outside the family. Thus the habit of dissection from early years came to be discontinued . . . it followed that the instruction became the poorer . . . the Art . . . was degenerating from one generation to the next. Thus too there arose a demand for memoranda to preserve knowledge . . . my contemporaries have little regard for the arts and sciences . . . and they no longer have practice from their early years.[57] . . . [anatomists] have elaborated with great care the part of anatomy that is completely useless to physicians. . . . Perched high on a professorial chair a man can say . . . things to his pupils without being able to instruct them in the actual practice of the art . . . [my work] is not only for physicians but for philosophers.[58]

Galen's concept of the worth of medicine is summed up as follows:

> The excellent state of health results from good care, as well as one can tell, and sickness comes from imperfect care, and we should attempt to correct inclemencies of health by making more moist those states which are too dry, and drying those conditions which are too moist. Likewise we get rid of overabundance of those states which are too warm and we encourage the abundance of those states which are too cold.[59]

To the modern reader, Galen's statement of the method and purpose of medicine may appear hopelessly confused and permeated with a kind of fuzzy double-talk. This common judgement is grossly incorrect and highly unfair to ancient medical concepts. We must first recognize that Galen had firmly rejected the accidental, atomistic concepts of medicine advanced by

Asclepiades.[60] His philosophy is one seeking purpose in the structures he observes, that is a teleology which was understandable given the general mood of his age.[61] The dead end appears to be reached as Galen is forced to rely upon the 'doctrine of humours' to treat patients and explain observed medical phenomena.[62] Like Roman imperial culture as a whole, Galenic medicine represents the consolidation of the best segments of Greek, Hellenistic, and Roman traditions. After his death, the creative process of discussion and dissection tapered off into treatises which took Galen at his word.[63]

The individual schooled in Greek philosophy easily understood Hellenistic medical theories, but their application to practical medicine was vague and often tediously prolix at best. In fusing many of the approaches, Eclecticism seemed to add to the confusion. Conscious experiment did not form an important part of the physician's concept of his work, and usually he was interested in mastering the great work which had preceded him. Galen provided the last gasp of creative endeavour in Roman medicine, but he too worked in the surroundings of Greek philosophy and an age saturated by magic and pseudo-science. Although Galen was not a great intellect, in a sense he represented that prodigious appetite for hard work and honest effort which characterized Pliny.[64]

CHAPTER IV

CATO AND THE MEDICAL
ENCYCLOPEDISTS

ALONGSIDE THE THEORETICAL 'SCHOOLS' of medicine in the late
Republic and the early Empire, there is a considerable body of
medical literature which is more specifically Roman. Not only is
it written in Latin, but also it is addressed to the practical needs of
the Roman landowners. This type begins with the work of Cato
the Elder and continues on through the encyclopedists.

In his attempt to preserve Roman attitudes for medical treatment on the farm, Cato performed the difficult task of setting
down known treatment in a reasonably accessible manner. The
Roman world had become broader by Cato's day, and restlessness
with traditional values became commonplace.[1] Hannibal had
come and gone and the tone of Roman society no longer was that
of the farm and the farmer's mentality. The late Republic was
dominated by the Great City and urban factors determined
Roman response to growing problems. Nevertheless, the Roman
approach to medical problems retained its simplistic character,
and Cato set a pattern of compilation followed by Varro and
Celsus. The extension of Roman supremacy was coupled with the
extension of Roman intellectual views.

Cato had a rustic suspicion of those professing sophisticated
knowledge, and he quickly observed the weaknesses of Greek
theoretical medicine as it had come to the Romans. He was a
blunt critic of the sham he saw in Hellenism, and he combined his
native genius of versatility with a narrow patriotism. Cato
expressed an anti-aristocratic bias, particularly against the Hellen-
ized cliques in Roman politics after the Roman victory over

Philip V in the Second Macedonian War. He recognized the contributions of Greek literature, but rejected the rhetorical flourishes commonplace in his day. His *Origines* did away with emphasis on the individual heroes in history, and his *On Agriculture* promotes the Roman concept of self-sufficiency in all intellectual matters of worth to a Roman. Cato affected to despise learning, but he was a prolific writer. His relation with Greek thought is a complex of reaction, rejection, borrowing, admiration, and disgust.

Roman encyclopedism is usually castigated for being unoriginal copy-work from Greek or Hellenistic sources.[2] Cicero is cited as taking Greek philosophy and popularizing it for the Roman lay reader.[3] Yet Cicero's translations supplied Latin with new words, and by the age of Varro, Cicero and Celsus, that Roman public had exhibited an interest in matters other than the direct history of an Ennius or a Cato.[4] The skill with which Cicero adapted Greek terms for the Latin context speaks eloquently for his creative synthesis which required a good amount of original thought.[5] Cato, Varro, Vitruvius, and most particularly Celsus, show the quality of clear Roman synthesis.[6] One of the finest poems in Latin, the *De rerum natura* by Lucretius, brings this ability of the Roman mind into even clearer focus.[7] The purpose of the encyclopedia in classical literature was not that of a modern encyclopedia, but it meant the gathering of books concerned with several subjects of practical value for edification *en kuklo*. The Roman encyclopedia thereby achieved a system of the known arts.[8] Within the structure of the Roman encyclopedia, changes were signalled in Roman ideas of medical theory and practice. Major authors in this genre include Varro, Celsus, and Pliny the Elder, but other writers show similar tendencies. Cato provides us with the earliest Latin effort at medical encyclopedism.

The Romans were slow to adapt Hellenistic medical ways, but they were quick to borrow the generally useful, and slower to accept the value of the generally theoretical. The practice of an Asclepiades had far less effect upon Roman values in medicine than did the writings of Cato. Cato was one of the Roman intellectuals who ostensibly led the fight against Greek influence in the late Republic, and whose invective would be mirrored in Juvenal.[9] Cato's reaction to Greek medicine was outwardly pointed and negative, but he foreshadowed the amalgamation in the complex intellectual world of Varro, Cicero, Vitruvius, Celsus, and Pliny.

Cato presents a knotty puzzle to the modern reader. On the one hand, he advises his son absolutely to avoid Greeks and their medicine, yet he is proud he has consulted Greek books on medicine.[10] There may be a jealousy felt by the native professional (as the Romans thought of him) for the all-too-successful foreigner who approaches problems with new ideas. The social and cultural history of the late Republic allows us to make a reasonable conjecture about the apparent schizophrenia and xenophobia of Cato. He lived through the Second Punic War and was talented in legal matters, and this ability brought him to the attention of Lucius Valerius Flaccus.[11] Under his patronage, Cato was launched on his political career. He reached the consulship in 195 BC, and served with distinction in the war against Antiochus III, but associated with the faction opposed to the philhellenism of the Scipios. Cato represented Roman attempts at reconstruction of venerated moral, social, and economic values in the face of growing Hellenistic influence, and his writing was a direct result of his Latin concept. His is the literary stimulus which directed further development of Latin prose.

Cato had a double-sided image to project to the public of his day: he wanted to be known as one of the group of poverty-stricken farmers who had become politically successful, and he wanted to be the champion of the Antihellenists. The powerful image obscures the modern (as well as the ancient) view of Cato and how he conducted himself regarding Greeks and Greek learning. Plutarch is deceived by the propaganda shield, thinking Cato learned Greek towards the end of his life. Later, Plutarch seems to have second thoughts as he contradicts himself by saying that Cato studied under the Pythagorean philosopher, Nearchus of Tarentum, after the fall of that city in 209 BC.[12] Plutarch had problems with Cato, much as does the modern reader, and consequently Plutarch bungles the chronology of Cato's early career.[13] Probably Cato learned some colloquial Greek while serving in Sicily under Marcellus from 214 to 210 BC.[14] Plutarch notes that Cato could have spoken in Greek to the Athenians, had he wished, on his mission in 191 BC.[15] His acquaintance, or rather knowledge, of Greek literature is illustrated a number of times.[16] The advice given by Cato to his son,[17] whether or not Pliny records the actual words or what Cato was supposed to have said, did not have real effect. Marcus absorbed enough Hellenism from his father to marry into one of the Hellenizing families.[18] The facts and Cato's official pose were two different matters.

Cato's extant work, *On Agriculture*, shows the paradox. Probably Cato wrote his manual without consultation of Hellenistic handbooks on agriculture,[19] but he was well aware of Hellenistic organization of agricultural technique.[20] Cato hoped, by setting down what was known of agricultural and medical knowledge in Italy, to show to his age that Romans could produce works of importance in these areas too. Cato's Hellenization was apparent on his own farms. He practised scientific plantation agriculture and used slave gangs on the Sicilian method.[21] Cato further revealed his Hellenization by supervising the building of the first basilica of the Hellenic style in Rome, in the year he was censor.[22]

Cato's importance in the history of medicine in Rome is wedded to his importance to Latin literature. Earlier attempts to write history for Romans were made in Greek by such as Fabius Pictor,[23] but Cato made the important innovation of using the Latin language as his means of reproducing what might be useful. The result, as Varro and Celsus would show, was that the Romans created a literature that took some stylistic tips from the Greek, but kept Latin as the expression of their thoughts on their own terms. The further history of both historical production and medical writings demonstrates similar paths. The later successful histories of Rome written for a Greek-speaking public were written by such as Polybius, Diodorus, Appian, Cassius Dio, Zosimus, and Procopius, and Latin efforts sport such names as Sallust, Caesar, Tacitus, and Suetonius. With the exception of Celsus, later efforts in the written history of Roman medicine were to be put down in Greek, and Rufus, Aretaeus, and Galen stand in the tradition of Greek writing for Greek readers. Of course educated Romans would speak of 'our two languages',[24] but Latin and its blunt approaches absorbed some of the Greek techniques in what Toynbee terms 'the creation of a Greek-style literature in Latin'.[25]

Cato stood at the juncture in time when the Roman aristocrat could speak with authority in medical matters, and the time when new knowledge from many sources was making the collective experience of the *Pater familias* inadequate. Underneath the acid against the Greeks, Cato indicated Roman shrewdness in creative adaptation. He was well aware of some of the advantages of the Hellenistic methods.[26] Plutarch may realize this, but the venom preserved by Pliny obscures the correct picture.[27] Possibly Cato's wrath was the result of a bitter personal experience with such as Archagathus, and reinforced his natural suspicion of Greek doctors. Pliny took the symbol of Cato as an old Roman, stripped him of un-Roman characteristics, and eulogized the result.[28]

Cato shows influences from the Hellenistic world, but the Roman environment altered these patterns. Although Plutarch's story of Cato studying with Nearchus at Tarentum is chronologically unsound, the tradition of Pythagoreanism sifting into Rome is worth consideration. This was a gradual matter, and is normally ignored in consideration of the intellectual revolution in the late Republic. Cato was affected by ideas from Magna Graecia, and his 'Roman' household medicine reflects these influences.[29] Thrown in with many Greek notions are native Italian folk themes which give Cato's work the Latin cast noted in Chapter I. Cato was indebted to Hellenistic and Carthaginian ideas and his work set a style of amalgamation for Latin scientific efforts.

After Cato comes Varro in the last years of the Roman Republic and, though his work stands outside strictly medical writings, his encyclopedia is important for the reasons that Cato was for his age. Again, borrowing, adaptation, and Roman moulding of Hellenistic models are clear. Varro takes the course suggested by Cato and makes the Roman farm the centre of his discussion, and includes all the fields of knowledge the Roman *Pater familias* was expected to know. Medicine figures in the discussion as it did in the work of Cato. In his enthusiasm for Italy and its productivity, Varro says candidly he is borrowing material from Cato.[30] Varro and Vergil both make use of Hellenistic illustration infused with Roman customs, and their thoughts indicate that Cato was a part of this past which had recognized the value of certain of the Hellenistic models.[31]

Varro notes the importance of a trained physician at given times on the farm, but usually 'an intelligent shepherd can attend to medical needs.' This important assertion of Roman reliance upon a method of medicine requiring little specialized training is a reflection of Cato, and Varro restates the idea several times. 'The shepherd should keep written down other diseases and symptoms,' and the manager of the flock 'should keep written directions concerning the remedies to be used for the various diseases [of the flock] and for wounds that they suffer.' The herdsman received instructions from his master, and Varro defines what he means by medical treatment. He states, 'all the matters relating to the health of men and cattle can be taken care of without the services of a physician, and all illnesses can be treated by the chief herdsman who keeps instructions in writing.'

Another section of Varro's treatise outlines the Roman concept of health and the role of medicine in the ideal. In the mould of Cato, Varro speaks of 'profit and pleasure' as what a farmer should strive to attain. On his ideal farm, 'land which is more healthy [*salubrior*] has more value, as there the profit [*fructus*] is certain.' 'The risk [of dealing with unhealthy locations] can be diminished by skilled understanding [*scientia*]. Although health is not under our control but is a result of climate and the soil, and within the power of nature, yet many matters [pertaining to health] rest with us. We are able through attentive investigations to lessen the unhealthy effects.' Varro continues by describing how a skilled farmer must lay out his buildings as well as note the exposure of doors and windows. The Roman concept of Greek medical skill slips in as Varro mentions Hippocrates: 'Did not the famous physician Hippocrates save not only one farm but numerous towns during a great pestilence through his skilled understanding [*scientia*]?'[32]

This understanding of medicine and its usefulness was not in the Hellenistic pattern, in which a specialized training was necessary to be educated in medical matters.[33] Although the Roman adapted many of the Hellenistic methods for his own use as far as was practical, he felt his intelligence and understanding would suffice in many problems. Medicine was thought of in terms connected with the traditional *Pater familias*. Perhaps a remark of Pliny[34] indicates that the Hellenistic theories were not understood by the Roman, or they were ignored in favour of direct results. The Roman drew no distinction between the theory and practice of medicine. Hellenistic physicians, however, acknowledged a difference between empirical and advanced study.[35]

Vitruvius in architecture and Celsus in medicine are excellent examples of a Roman willingness to adapt the generally practical, and refusal to admit speciality in a theoretical sense. This tendency carried its tradition into the late Empire. The Roman attempt at practical extraction degenerated into rag-tag compilations resembling folk recipes.[36] The Roman government encouraged Greek doctors to settle in Rome, but, in the age of Augustus and Tiberius, the outstanding concepts of medicine were voiced by Vitruvius and Celsus in Latin.

Vitruvius' work is a compilation of Hellenistic architectural theory combined with Roman practical experience.[37] Vitruvius gives numerous examples of the Roman approach to medicine as it applies to the training and practice of architecture. The dichotomy in the Roman mind between the theoretical and its application is firm. As a Roman, he announces the usefulness of medicine by noting that the architect should know something of medicine, because of the problems in architecture relating to climate, air, the matter of health related to various sites, and the qualities of water. 'For if one does not consider these factors, the health of a dwelling cannot be assured.' He continues his discussion with a garbled atomistic medical analysis showing the Roman empirical approach. A sceptical, observational view of life is prominent. Vitruvius shows he is acquainted with Hellenistic works as he touches on the problems of judging distances and depth accurately, but he adds his own doubts. 'An appearance', he says, 'may result from impact of images, or the effusion of rays from the eye, as the physicists tell us . . . sight can give us false impressions.'[38]

Fact by association with known phenomena is important for Vitruvius. He describes the qualities of healing springs:

. . . rocks of lava, which neither iron nor fire can alone dissolve, split into pieces and dissolve when heated with fire and sprinkled with vinegar. Hence, since we see these things taking place before our very eyes, we may infer that on the same principle even patients with the stone may, in the nature of things, be cured in like manner by means of acid waters on account of the sharpness of the potion.[39]

Some springs [being acid] . . . when used as drinks, have the power of breaking up stones in the bladder, which form in the human body.[40]

Roman empiricism, as Vitruvius expresses it, shows that the educated Roman did not accept Hellenistic ideas without question. The later handbook tradition may have been the result of uncritical use of these writers, but it was not true of such authors as Varro, Vitruvius, and Celsus.[41] Within the scope of learning of the well-educated Roman, medical theory is used as far as it possibly may apply to everyday situations. Sound reason characterizes the adaptation.

Vitruvius' *On Architecture* is a guide for the Roman architect, but it also denotes the Roman mental ability in many fields of intellectual endeavour. Medical observations were a part of the Latin scientific literature in the early Empire.[42] The high quality of Latin in Varro and Celsus excites admiration, and the medical concepts of the Roman citizen, glimpsed in Cicero, attest to the general upgrading and depth of Roman learning in this period.[43]

Around the figure of the Roman encyclopedist, Celsus, rages one of the more heated topics in the study of medicine in antiquity. He is called either a physician who 'practised medicine', or merely a Roman compiler of a Hellenistic medical handbook.[44]

There is truth in both viewpoints since medicine in the early
Roman Empire was a composite of Hellenistic medical theory
and Roman practical approaches. Celsus, termed by his eulogists
Cicero medicorum, is our best example in Latin literature of the
application of the theory and practice of medicine by a superbly
educated Roman aristocrat with a keen mind.

Celsus' status as an authority on medicine—as the Romans conceived of it—is unquestionable. Columella uses him as a major
source for his work, and many of the remarks on medical care on
the farm are from Celsus.[45] Columella regards Celsus as a learned
expert on the whole of natural science.[46] Quintilian reflects this
when he terms Celsus knowledgeable in rhetoric, agriculture,
war, and medicine.[47] Pliny lists Celsus among his *auctores*, but
not among the physicians, and Celsus stands as a 'doctor' who
'practised' as a Roman within the concept of the *Pater familias*.[48] As
the evidence indicates, Celsus did not practise medicine in the
Hellenistic definition, but certainly he was a doctor in the traditional Roman sense.[49]

The loud cries of resentment for the Hellenistic physicians,
voiced by Cato and Pliny, have their quieter counterpart in
Celsus. Celsus notes the tradition of vivisection from Alexandria,
argues the merits of the practice, and rejects it as barbarous. In the
Roman view, the Hellenistic theories confused more than they
cured, although Celsus writes with great respect for the Greek
theoretical achievement.[50] He deals with problems in a succinct,
straightforward manner, and Hellenistic theory is presented as an
indication that this is what 'the learned physicians from the east
have to say about it'.[51] He feels he can extract what is important
from Hellenistic theory and put it to good use as a Roman
medicus.[52] Within the Roman household, Hellenistic doctors were
most often slaves or freedmen, and their function presents a
paradox to the modern observer.[53] Celsus says these individuals
can give insight into medical problems, and they handle cases a
Roman *medicus* avoids, but they practise medicine on a different
level than would a Roman.[54]

The mood of *On Medicine* is strongly Latin, and the work is a
great product of Roman synthesis. *On Medicine* performs the same

service for Roman readers of medicine that Cicero did for philosophical writing. Celsus translates many Greek terms into Latin and supplies them with a proper context in a well-balanced consideration of the whole of medicine as it was known in the first century. It is not surprising that Vesalius, in the sixteenth century, was enthusiastic over Cicero and Celsus, and sought to use both styles in his monumental *De Fabrica*.[55]

Celsus speaks about the use of good medical habits, and he voices concern lest the Romans may ignore the useful. He hints that the context of the time makes it imperative the Romans use their reason to determine the best way of living.

But the frail, of whom there are a large proportion of town dwellers and who are, for the most part, fond of learning, must take great care, so that attention [to these problems] might restore that which the aspect of their general health or of their home or of their study would take away.[56]

For the person who has been occupied during the day, whether in public or private matters, should designate some part of the day for the care of his body. His first concern in this regard should be exercise, which ought always to precede the eating of food. The exercise should be greater for him who has worked less and considered well, and it should be lighter for him who is tired and who has thought less during the day.[57]

Sexual intercourse neither should be avidly desired, nor should it be feared very much. Rarely performed, it revives the body, performed frequently, it weakens. However, since nature, and not number should be considered in frequency, with consideration of age and the state of the body, sexual union is recognized as not harmful when it is followed by neither apathy nor pain.[58]

Celsus explains what the Roman thinks is the purpose of medicine, as defined from current Hellenistic medicine and its application.

A healthy man, who is both strong and his own master,

ought not to place himself under any arbitrary rules, nor should he have a need for a doctor nor for an iatrolipta.[59] His sort of life should give him variety. He should sometimes be in the country, sometimes in the city, more often should he be on a farm. He should sail, hunt, rest from time to time, but more frequently exercise his body. While inactivity weakens the body, work makes it strong; the former gives an early old age, and the latter promotes an extended youth.[60]

Thus I infer that the physician who does not know the particular characteristics of a disease ought to consider its general symptoms. And he who is able to come to know particular characteristics ought not to neglect the broad characteristics, but he should emphasize them. And therefore, since the acquaintance of both by the physician should be equally emphasized, it is more useful that the physician be a friend rather than a stranger. Therefore, I would return to my theme. I believe that the medical art should be rational, and to gain instruction from evident causes, and with all obscure causes rejected from the art, but not from the reflection of the skilled physician. Thus to lay open the bodies of men while they yet live is both cruel and needless, but for all those learning the art it is necessary to study the bodies of the dead. For they ought to know position and arrangement, which the cadaver shows better than would a living man who is wounded. As for the rest, which can be learned only from the living, it will be shown in the actual care of the wounded in a somewhat slower but in a far more gentle fashion.[61]

Celsus' attitudes towards the Hellenistic schools of medicine are ambivalent, as many references in the *Prooemium* and elsewhere attest.[62] Celsus, the Roman physician, practising in the tradition of Cato in the role of *Pater familias*, found the usual all-knowing attitudes were insufficient to cope with new situations in the early Empire. Celsus attempted to solve this problem in an expected Roman manner. He set down what he thought best of medical practice in his day. Celsus took his thoughts from both the native Latin tradition and the Hellenistic schools. As a good, sceptical Roman, he weeded out the obviously faulty in the Hellenistic methods.

Celsus was influenced by Asclepiades and Heracleides of Tarentum, but only slightly through recipes and their usefulness.[63] Celsus' own concepts of medicine retained their Roman tone. If the charge of copyist-compiler can be hurled against him, the books of recipes might provide reason for accusation. Lists, however, do not allow an understanding of medicine, as Celsus points out.[64] He provides the recipes of drugs so that physicians within Roman tradition could use them with a greater degree of accuracy, but not be ignorant of their various properties.

Columella follows in the tradition of Cato and Varro, and his work resembles the easy style which distinguishes Celsus. His birthplace was in Spain, and Columella represents the Latinization of the western provinces.[65] The style of On Agriculture is pleasant, and would appeal to the country reader because Columella knows when not to be eloquent. In viewing the repetition by Columella of Varro's and Cato's agricultural encyclopedias, as well as some sections from Celsus' work on agriculture, we note the Roman tradition maintained in the face of massive Greek influence. The farm continues as the Roman's own. Medical references are easy enough to come by, provided that the intelligent Roman draws the proper conclusion from the Latin customs and the new ideas from the Hellenistic world. Although the motif of Columella is a Cato-like agriculture, the tone has changed considerably. Instead of the heartless assertions of Cato in regard to slaves, the humaneness and gentleness of the farmer, coupled with a love for the countryside, run as dual themes through the work of Columella. He notes sadly that slaves worked in chains and were kept cooped up at night in an underground prison, the *ergastulum*.[66] Varro, Celsus, and Columella would have Roman efficiency, but they were repelled and ashamed by the history of Roman brutality.

Pliny the Elder, in speaking about the curative powers of cabbage, admits his debt to the native Roman tradition, with Cato as its proponent.[67] Pliny shows a fantastic energy, at least in the amount of material that is represented in the *Natural History*. The same gentle, curious mood permeates Pliny's work as in Celsus and Columella. The characterization of Pliny, written some years after his death, shows him restless and always occupied in what the modern man calls antiquarianism.[68] Pliny indicates the Roman adeptness at synthetic intellectual structures at its best, and at its worst. Stahl may be correct in arguing that Pliny represents the tradition of Latin science as it survived in the west, but Pliny exhibited many of the excellent qualities of the Roman syncretic mind.

> It would be too lengthy a task to enumerate all the praises of the cabbage, more particularly as the physician Chrysippus has devoted a whole volume to the subject. . . . Cato, too, has not been more sparing in its praises than the others; and it will only be right to examine the opinions which he expresses in relation to it, if for no other reason than to learn what medicines the Roman people made use of for six hundred years.[69]

Pliny, however, has a certain facility for uncritical use of his material.

> And Cato recommends the urine of a person who has been living on a cabbage diet to be preserved, as, when it is warmed, it is a good remedy for diseases of the sinews. I will, however, here give the identical words in which Cato expresses himself on this point: 'If you wash little children with this urine,' says he, 'they will never be weak and puny.'[70]

Pliny uses some of his short excursions into the various fields of history of science to 'stand up to the Greeks' in favour of Roman ability.[71] According to Pliny, the practical knack of the Roman can give a better answer than can theoretical Greek speculation. Pliny, as the manner of his death would suggest, would go and look whenever possible, and thereby draw his own conclusions. He speaks to us today as an example of the indefatigable amateur who devoted his life to collecting interesting facts for the edification of his fellows. His usefulness was recognized from the time his books appeared until the dawn of modern pharmacology and medicine in the late Renaissance. His relation to his time, intellectually, is far too complex to analyse in a few words, but many similarities exist between Cato and Pliny. In many ways, Cato was an admirable person, but he was narrow and cruel on some of the most important intellectual questions of his day. Pliny was not narrow or cruel, but his concept of *Romanitas* was essentially the same as Cato's. In medical problems, Cato and Pliny represent a negative position which has given rise to disgust in readers ever since the Middle Ages.

In sum, the broadening of the Roman concept of medicine, in the exercise of encyclopedic medicine expressed in Latin, has two strands: one is observed as the finest of synthetic processes, with an adaptability and a soundness of judgement greatly to be admired. Celsus, Varro, and Vitruvius show the Roman mind at work in the new Empire, forming a fresh intellectual world with their native ability and the modification of multitudinous foreign influences. The second strand is seen in Cato and Pliny, who speak of the tradition of Roman medicine as a series of recipes, and this variety of folk medicine lives on in our own day.[72] The medical practice fashioned by Celsus incorporated that which was outwardly sound from the Hellenistic speculations as well as Roman practical productivity, and made it into a manageable, unified whole.

CHAPTER V

MEDICAL PRACTICE AND
THE ROMAN ARMY

SINCE CELSUS WAS a Roman aristocrat who practised medicine in the tradition of the noble household, we note that our evidence for the practice of medicine among the Romans comes through indirect method, as the Romans did not admit the 'speciality' of medicine on the part of a Roman practitioner. None the less, we possess specific evidence on one segment of Roman society, giving us an exact view of the Roman concepts of medicine. The practice of medicine in the Roman army is fairly well lit through epigraphy, but often the legionary *medicus* is misconstrued in modern accounts.

Most histories of medicine make reference to the remarkable state of medicine in the Roman legions, but the literature on the topic is surprisingly limited.[1] Skilled medical practitioners are usually depicted accompanying the legion on its campaigns, and a glance at the available evidence seems to leave little doubt that the legion was well-supplied with *medici*. Yet once the modern observer has probed beneath appearances transmitted by the numerous inscriptions found throughout the Empire, and analysed what is meant by 'skilled' care in the legions, he recognizes that factors making up Celsus' approach to medicine are also valid for the practice of medicine in the army. The legionary ranks reflected aspects of Roman aristocratic medicine, and the *medicus* who appears in the legion bears close resemblance to the *medicus* of Celsus, Varro, and Pliny.

Sources for the development of Roman medical practice in the Republican legion are sparse and often subject to conjecture.

Those authors who tell us something of the early history of Rome and her arduous conquest of the Italian peninsula have few references to medical problems in the phalanx-legion as it evolved in the early Republic. There was little provision for the wounded, and medical care was minimal. The evolution of medical practice in the legions resembled closely the development of medicine among the Romans as a whole. Medicine functioned to keep the soldiers as healthy as possible, and the crude medical care that existed in the legions was practised by the soldiers upon one another, as we would expect citizens to do in Roman civilian life. Military medicine sought to get the soldier back into battle as quickly as possible, and the more seriously wounded were left to fend for themselves. The consul took care of some of the wounded as far as he was able, but a generalized attitude prevailed which allowed the legionaries to be unworried about medical aid.[2]

A good general sometimes billeted his seriously wounded legionaries in a friendly town or fortress.[3] Within the sanctuary, the wounded soldier was dependent upon his fellows for help, or he received care from well-disposed townsmen or their wives in the traditional mode of the aristocratic household. The soldiers often commanded as much skill as their benefactors, and both practised a sort of 'folk' medicine, resembling Cato's prescriptions or Varro's general principles.[4]

Before Hellenistic influence, the Republican legion did not contain any medical services, distinguished as such, other than the soldiers themselves, or the consul, who were deemed skilled in their primitive care.[5] The problem of the wounded, however, was not of great importance to the Roman legion provided it won its battles. Generally the legion fought on its own terms in conditions judged by its consul favourable for winning, and the techniques of retreat developed in the manipular legion lessened the incidence of wounded even in defeat. The victorious army in antiquity normally did not lose too many men, but those who lost—fighting in the usual phalanx formation—lost everything.[6]

Hellenistic influence upon the Roman legion was limited, but as the Romans came to know the practices within the Hellenistic phalanx, the consul and his staff adopted a procedure common

among professional generals of the Hellenistic world. A personal
physician often accompanied the general on the battlefield and
attended to his wants and hurts.[7] The consul valued the doctor for
the encouragement he gave to the wounded, but the physician
was not considered as useful as a skilled general who could not
only 'hearten the wounded but also cause them to stand again'.[8]
The physician's equipment was simple, consisting of drugs and
probably a few surgical tools.[9] His function was usually limited to
treatment with his drugs,[10] but on occasion he served the general
as a surgeon.[11]

Onasander leaves us with the distinct impression that the
'wounded' treated by the physicians present in the army were of the
higher ranks.[12] Before a definite reference from Cicero,[13] there is
little indication that the common soldiers had access to medical
care. The soldiers of the higher ranks, who were of aristocratic extraction, had 'refreshment retreats' in their tents to which they re-
tired when they became tired or wounded. The Romans regarded
the 'retreat' as a portable relaxation point rather than a special place
to go for the treatment of wounds.[14]

The Roman consul borrowed some of the methods recorded in
Onasander and Xenophon,[15] and adopted them with Roman
forthrightness. Some of the troops functioned as a medical staff as
the need arose, particularly to help their fellows. The professional
physicians were individuals who probably were of the consul's
household staff and who functioned in his personal service as they
did at home.[16] Medical skill was part of the consul's collective
experience, and he was often a skilled wound-dresser in his own
right. Such knowledge stemmed from long years in the aristocratic household or in the legions.[17]

Cicero tells us the experienced soldier was confident of treatment on the battlefield, but the novice despaired at the slightest
hurt.[18] Silius Italicus notes the soldier expected someone to come
and bind up his wounds, and Caesar indicates that soldiers had
their wounds dressed.[19] Before Cicero, we have no proof of care
for the common soldier, yet his use of *medicus* shows his function
was customary, and his fellow-legionaries sought him out.
Cicero's imprecise language leaves the modern reader with the

supposition that the *medicus* was just another soldier, but one who was judged experienced among the legionaries in problems of wound-dressing.[20] Usually anyone who appeared as if he knew something of medicine received the designation *medicus*, and Apollo-*medicus* commanded a large following with a series of quasi-medical sayings.[21]

The Hellenistic literary tradition provided the Romans with a clear stereotype of the military physician, and he appears from time to time with a specialized function related to the care of the commander. In Quintus Smyrnaeus, the attendant doctors cleanse wounds, stitch them together when they can, and swab them liberally with soothing ointments, 'which had been bequeathed from ancient times'.[22] The salves furnished the major help the physician gave to the wounded,[23] but the doctor received his power from the gods as he anointed wounds.[24] The doctor also had skill to brew up poisons, which could be disguised as curing potions,[25] and possessed a certain talent in surgery.[26] The physician feared a real operation and he was not certain of its results.[27] Poisoned missiles baffled the doctor and he watched helplessly as the soldiers died from trifling wounds.[28]

Vergil sums up the inveterate figure of the military physician as the Roman thought of him in the first century BC, and the sketch resembles that of Quintus Smyrnaeus and Quintus Rufus. The literary image links well with the evidence we possess for both the civilian and military modes of medicine in the late Republic and the early Empire.

> At this point, Iapis, the son of Iasus, came up: this man was especially dear to Apollo, who, seized by intense passion for him, had delightedly offered him his own arts, his own powers of divination, of music, of shooting the swift-flying arrow. Iapis, to lengthen the life of a father desperately ill, elected the knowledge of healing herbs, the science of medicine choosing to practise an art which has little *réclame*, in obscurity.[29]

Vergil on occasion gives clues to the common attitude about a soldier's troubles, and the military man received admiration for

the amount of physical punishment he could take. Vergil echoes
some of the heartless statements that strike the modern reader in
the fragments of Ennius.[30]

Caesar has passages which allow us to determine whether or not
an official medical corps was available to the Roman legionary.
His regard for the safety and well-being of his trusted legions is
apparent as he writes. Concern for individuals serving under his
standards marks Caesar as one of the great leaders in history, and
a passage from the *Gallic War*, which relates to our discussion,
emphasizes his attention.

> One of the sick men who had been left behind with the
> guard was Publius Sextius Baculus. He served under Caesar
> as a senior centurion, and has already been mentioned in
> regard to previous battles. He had already been five days
> without food. Now unsure about his own safety, and that
> of the others, he went forth from his tent unarmed. . . .
> Sextius fell unconscious as he was seriously wounded, and he
> was saved just barely by being dragged from the scene from
> hand to hand.[31]

Caesar praises the man's valour, and eulogy of this kind is
repeated throughout the *Gallic War*.[32] It seems odd, however,
that although Caesar reports numbers of the wounded and the
condition of some of the wounded, he fails to account for how
they might have been treated.[33] Jacob argues that, since Caesar
does not bother to talk of this matter, the wounded were taken
care of by a medical corps that Caesar took for granted.[34] A
sounder conclusion would be that there was a kind of *de facto*
medical service of soldier-*medici* which obviated notice.

An official medical service was not a part of the Roman consul's
planning on the field of battle. The account given by Plutarch of
the disaster at Carrhae points this up sharply.[35] With an elaborate
expedition such as Crassus prepared against Parthia, a medical staff
would have been included if it had been customary to have an
official service on the battlefield. Again we can note that the
generals supplied themselves with physicians who attended to
their personal needs.[36] Caesar recognized the value of billeting his

wounded in a safe spot so that they might return to battle, and his system of evacuation of his wounded shows considerable foresight.[37] The major characteristic of the references that Caesar gives us about his sick and wounded is one of praise for the endurance of his troops, and great hints of the typical cold-blooded, 'stoic' attitude of the Roman legionary.

Thus by the end of the Republic, Roman military medicine was modelled to a certain degree upon precedents common in the Greek armies of the Hellenistic period. The consul and the noble elements of the legion supplied themselves with personal medical care, but the legionary was left in the care of the *medici*.[38] The superb discipline of the Roman legion and its winning record kept the usual incidence of wounded low, but the legionary, like his enemies, suffered from the devastations of disease until the use of the *valetudinarium* and sanitary measures became commonplace in the Empire.[39]

Inscriptions from the Empire, as well as further literary references, indicate the unofficial basis of medical care in the legions. In speaking of the *primorum ordinum* as being a select group of century commanders whom he used as an informal consultation committee, Caesar provides a key to explain the often occurring inscriptional *medicus ordinarius*.[40] Since Caesar's council was one of men taken from the ranks and distinctly one of an informal nature, the *medicus ordinarius*, *medicus cohortis*, and the *medicus legionis* functioned on the same basis. The inscriptions show that this position was one of great respect, but that the individual so named was first a soldier in his duties, not a physician.[41] It is to the Romans' credit that they recognized the need for such a service, but the solution was not a medical corps whereby trained physicians became a part of the army. The response to the problem of proper care for the sick and the wounded in the legions took the form that the Roman would understand and he thought that it was effective for the need as it was demonstrated. The wounded were cared for, as far as possible, on the field, and the transportable sick were placed in *valetudinaria* along with the more severely wounded. The Romans clearly distinguished in the legions between the treatment of the 'sick' and the 'wounded'.

Examples from the inscriptions and from archaeological excavation illustrate the approach. An inscription found in the vicinity of Hadrian's Wall tells in terse terms of gratitude what the soldiers of the first Tungrian Cohort felt for one Ancius Ingenuus, who had died at the age of twenty-five. His memorial tablet was embellished to an extent that might not be expected, and he is styled *medicus ordinarius*.[42] This indicates his status as one of the ranks, but his status of great respect among his fellow soldiers.[43] Compassion was as highly prized among the Roman legionaries as it is in any age. Titus Claudius Hymnus, *medicus legionis* to the XXI Claudia, is commemorated in a similar fashion.[44] The Cohors IV Praetoria gives us an interesting example of a *medicus cohortis* who erected a memorial to himself and to his dependants.[45] The tone of the inscription allows the modern viewer to observe what could be called 'scientific magic' in the taking of vows in connection with the function of the *medicus* in the legions. The Roman navy had its own variety of 'doctor', termed the *medicus duplicarius*, and his skill was limited.[46]

The great number of inscriptions indicate the *medicus* to be very common, particularly in the frontier posts. We can assume that the *medici* were on hand at most points to render what aid they could, and probably the newer *medici* learned their medicine from the 'senior' *medici* present in the legion.

As the Roman legion developed efficiency and learned to deal with isolated locations which made it impossible for the wounded to be evacuated to a safe Roman fort or allied town, it began to build *valetudinaria* which would serve this function. These structures were the Roman answer to isolation and proved to be an integral part of the *castra*, especially on the frontier.[47] Here the *medici*, experienced as they were in the wounds of war, treated their comrades. The legionary hospitals were carefully planned and show insight into drainage problems with regard to sanitary conditions.[48] Roman engineering skill is apparent and one must admire these islands of hope placed at the edge of the civilized world. Again it should be emphasized that the *valetudinaria* argue for the medical care of the sick as the Roman thought of them in contradistinction from the wounded. They indicate that the Roman

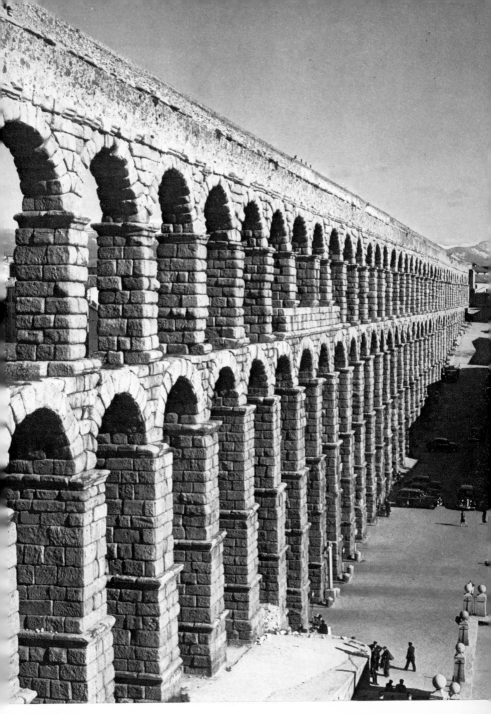

15 Roman aqueduct at Segovia, Spain. This is a good example of the cross valley construction justly famous from existing examples (*see* Fig. 12).

16, 17 Two examples of the medieval transmission of ancient medical concepts. *Below*, an illustration of the Celsan operation for bladder stones (*vide* Celsus VII, 26). The technique of the operation is essentially the same as described in the first century AD by Celsus. The present illustration is from a North Italian ms. of *c.* 1300 of Rolandus Parmensis, *Chirurgia* III, 34. *Opposite*, an illustration of the techniques and divisions of uroscopy. This fifteenth-century Byzantine example shows the patient handing the physician a urine sample. Below the figures are the classifications of urine shown in varying colours in the original ms. This diagnostic technique was well known in antiquity and Roman physicians elaborated upon Greek and Hellenistic methods (*vide* Galen, IX, 801; X, 947; XIX, 602-628; Rufus of Ephesus, 522-523. *Cf.* F. Henschen, *Medical History*, XIII, 1969, 190–92). From a ms. copy with Greek text of Theophilus Protospatharius, *On Urines*.

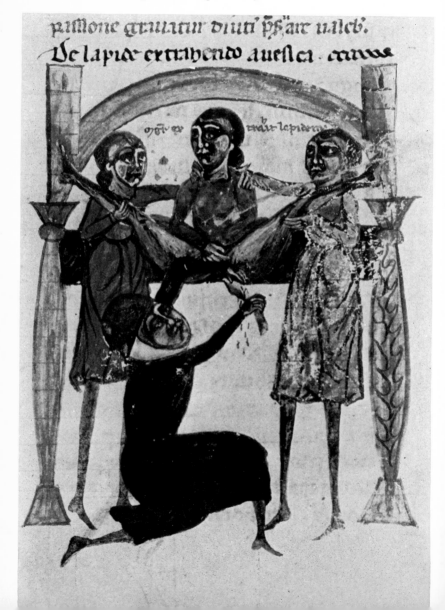

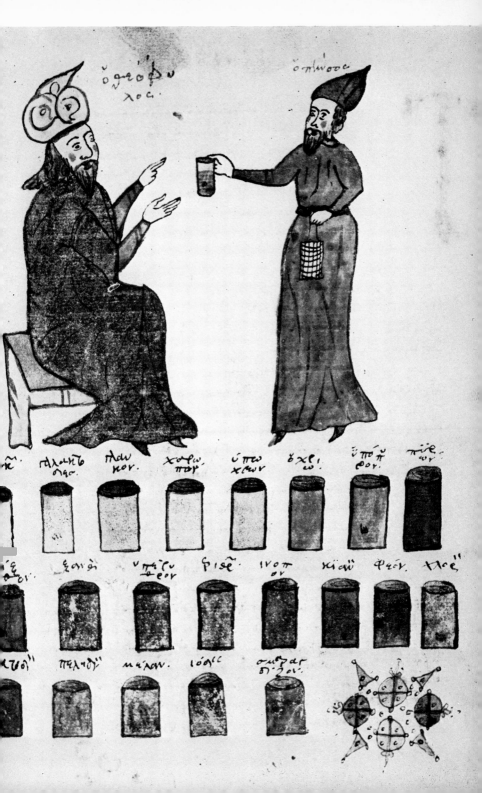

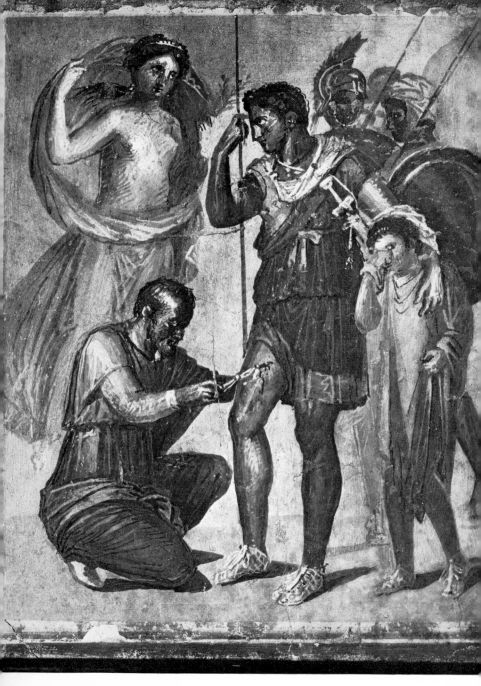

18 In this wall painting from Pompeii we see Iapis (?) removing an arrowhead from the leg of Aeneas. Apparently the instrument that he is using is a pair of pincers rather than the arrowscoop which is described by Celsus (*see* Fig. 9). Naples Museum.

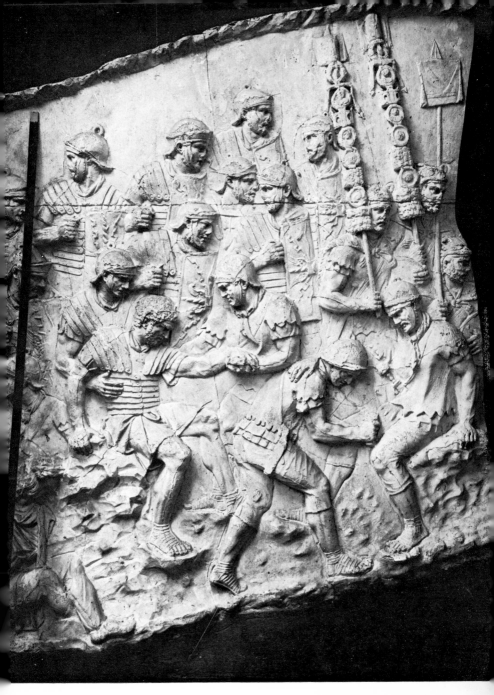

19 Detail from Trajan's Column, Rome. A legionary *medicus* is performing a rather
ill-defined operation on the right upper leg of one of his comrades. Note the
similarity in uniform between them suggesting that the *medicus* was an ordinary
legionary who functioned first as a soldier then as a medical orderly.

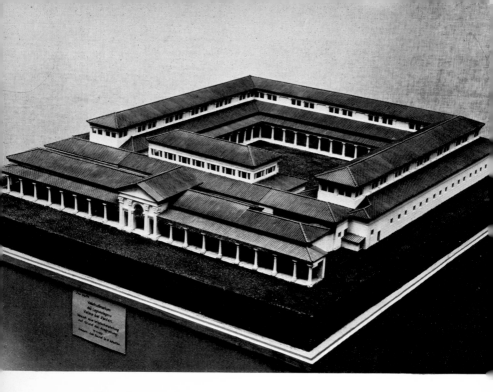

20, 21 Two views of a model reconstruction of the Roman legionary hospital at Vetera (modern Xanten). This reconstruction gives a large portico on a colonnade as the main entrance to the wards arranged around a colonnaded central court. The clerestory is hypothetical. Rheinisches Landesmuseum, Bonn.

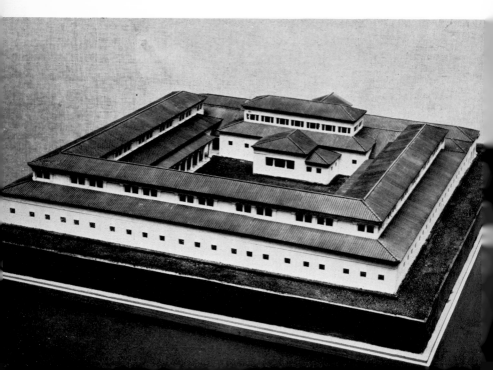

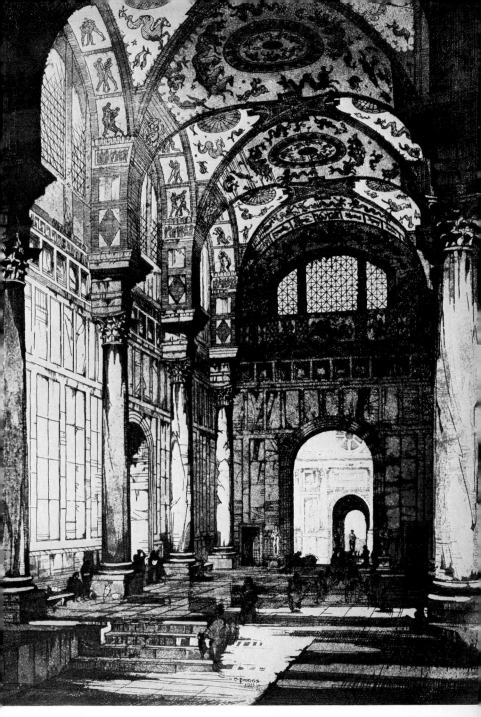

22 Reconstruction of the *frigidarium* of the Hadrianic Baths at Lepcis Magna. The hall was paved and panelled with marble and roofed by concrete cross-vaults. Note the immense height of the vault seen from the scale of the figures (*see* Fig. 6).

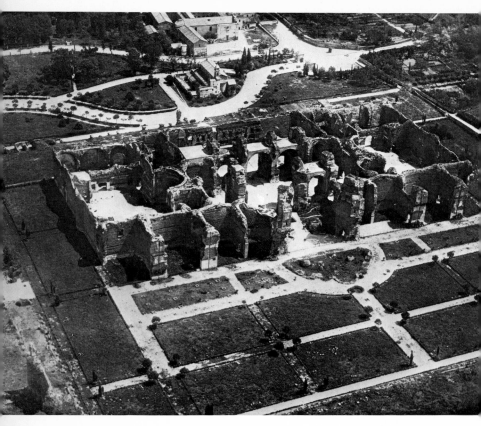

23 Aerial view of the Baths of Caracalla in Rome. This photograph clearly shows the area into which a bath building was divided (*cf.* Figs. 6 and 11). These baths are the most extensive remaining from the Roman Empire. Vitruvius goes into detail regarding the planning and siting of baths; Frontinus is similarly concerned about their supply of water.

army was following good military practice by providing a place
for the sick and the transportable wounded near to the source of
manpower need. In an age where geographical distances were
fantastic, this points to the element of genius inherent in Roman
military organization.

Literary evidence spanning the entire course of the Roman
Empire points firmly to the lack of an organization of an official
medical service which would administer to the common soldier.
In his praise of Tiberius, Velleius Paterculus reveals the presence of
medical care for the officers of the legions, but not for the common
soldier.

> And now for a detail which in telling may lack grandeur,
> but is most important by reason of the true and substantial
> personal qualities it reveals and also of its practical service—
> a thing most pleasant as an experience and remarkable for the
> kindness it displayed. Throughout the whole period of the
> German and Pannonian War there was not one of us, nor of
> those either above or below our rank, who fell ill without
> having his health and welfare looked after by Caesar with
> as much solicitude indeed as though this were the chief
> occupation of his mind, preoccupied though he was by his
> heavy responsibilities. There was a horsed vehicle for all those
> who needed it, his own litter was at the disposal of all, and I,
> among others, have enjoyed its use. Now his physicians, now
> his kitchen, now his bathing equipment, brought for this one
> purpose for himself alone, ministered to the comfort of all
> who were sick. All they lacked was their home and their
> domestic servants, but nothing else that friends at home
> could furnish or desire for them.[49]

Even the aristocrat was grateful for good medical care. The passage indicates that trained physicians available for the legion at
large were rare and that Tiberius followed the practice of the best
Roman generals. Such care was not usual and the soldiers received
the ministrations of the *medici* in their own ranks. In another
context Tacitus crisply notes the thankfulness of the soldiers

when Agrippina went among the wounded and acted as a nurse, dressing the wounds and giving clothing to those who needed it.[50] At another point Tacitus states bluntly that the soldiers took care of their own wounds and doctored one another.[51] The image of medicine in the legions shows no trained physician in attendance, and that the training of the *medici* consisted of experience with a common knowledge of anatomy and medicine in the day-to-day needs of the legion.

Celsus remarks that anatomy can be learned from the wounds of a soldier in battle and Galen says that the medical attendants in the German Wars were, like untrained Empirics, not to dissect the bodies of the dead German warriors to learn something more than they knew.[52] Celsus gives us a detailed account of missile injuries and this may show the level of skill attained by the best of the military *medici*.[53] From the evidence that we have of the *medicus*, he gathered his craft within the legion and was not a trained physician in either the Hellenistic fashion of Galen or in the Latinized fashion that Celsus suggested.[54]

The often-cited reliefs of a *medicus* treating the wounded, as depicted on Trajan's Column, reinforce the conclusions that the inscriptions and literary evidence give us. The *medici* treating the wounded on Trajan's Column are dressing superficial wounds and their dress is identical with that of the soldiers they are aiding.[55] Trajan's Column would thus bear out the general picture: the *medici* were those soldiers of a legion or of an auxiliary detachment who had demonstrated their capabilities for wound dressing and a primitive surgery, but who were not trained physicians.[56] This tradition reached back many centuries in Roman warfare. Whether or not the best of the Roman legionary *medici* consulted medical handbooks such as Celsus must remain theoretical.

Returning to further references from the literary sources, one notes the unofficial basis admitted in many cases. As time passed the soldiers seemed to have received less attention of the quality noted in the Early Empire, and the camp praefect was put in charge of what medical care they got.[57] Problems with camp followers posing as medical men are seen in the following:

Let the soldier be treated by a doctor without cost, let him give nothing to the soothsayers, let them spend their time in their quarters [*hospitiis*] in abstinence from sensual pleasures as if for religious reasons [*caste*].[58]

. . . those who are most knowledgeable in military matters are of the opinion that daily exercise contributes far greater health to the soldiers than do the physicians. . . .[59]

If trained physicians were present among the legions in the Later Empire, the type of medicine they practised seems to remind us of the repute of certain doctors often noted in authors of the Early Empire.[60] Galen tells us that he was summoned to give proper medical treatment at the front where little apparently existed—as he saw it. Galen notes that many doctors 'talk' medicine without proving their skill.[61]

Roman legionary medicine was an achievement, ranking with the *valetudinaria* the Romans established for the care of their sick and wounded. Like the *valetudinaria*, legionary medicine developed as the need called for it, and no formal pattern of medical training was ever instituted for the legionary *medicus* as he functioned within the army. The *medicus*, so often commemorated in our inscriptions, illuminates clearly the status of medicine as a defined activity among Romans as a whole. The soldiers learned what medicine they needed while in the service, and certain of the ranks became *medici* and ministered to the hurts of their fellows.

CHAPTER VI

THE ROMAN TECHNICAL
AND HYGIENIC ACHIEVEMENT

ROMAN DIRECTNESS led the Romans to excellent methods in solving immediate problems arising in disease and sanitation.[1] The military *valetudinaria* were not used in Roman society at large, but many of the techniques applied in the military health measures were reflected in the everyday life of the Roman citizen.[2] Roman agriculture showed remarkable insight into the problems of cultivation and use of fen land, and the Roman speculated upon the causes of sickness from the marsh with practical success.[3] In another response to practical need, surgeons in the Empire utilized the forms of medical tools coming to them from the Hellenistic world, but examples survive showing that the Roman improved a few of the Hellenistic prototypes from the school of experience.[4] In general concepts of public hygiene, the Romans had extraordinary ability for implementing the practical in such matters as water supply and sanitation, and keen discernment into the faults of medicine in its application.[5] Disparate authors, such as Celsus, Vitruvius, Pliny, Frontinus, Columella, Varro, and Vegetius, show the Roman concept of health interwoven with his usual life and the ordinary process of government in the Roman Empire.[6]

Properly a discussion of the Roman military *valetudinaria* belongs with consideration of Roman military medicine, but certain characteristics of the military response to practical need indicate the general quality of the Roman answer to public sanitation. It will be appropriate, therefore, to look at the *valetudinaria* in conjunction with Roman aqueducts and farm techniques.

The Romans developed military hospitals for the use of the wounded and ill legionaries, but the practice did not sift into Roman society as a whole.[7] Examples of hospitals on the *limes* are numerous, and their features prove the Roman ability to sense the workable in treatment of their sick.[8] At Inchtuthil in Scotland, excavators have uncovered the outlines of a large military hospital, having an area of 298 by 192 feet, and a superb drainage system from the hospital into one of the larger camp sewers.[9] The system drained the barrack roofs and the toilets in the offices of the centurions.[10] Other finds in Britain include the complex hospital system at Abergavenny in Monmouthshire, the extensive sewage works at Aldborough in West Riding, and sewers and numerous well-drained latrines at Leintwardine in Herefordshire. Bath construction at Wroxeter, Hedgerly in Buckinghamshire, Bath, Upper Thames Street in London, and Eccles in Kent exhibit careful planning similar to the *valetudinaria*.[11]

Hospital planning was an important part of legionary camp construction throughout the Empire. Switzerland, Germany, and North Africa, as well as Britain, provide well-preserved illustrations.[12] In the case of Lepcis Magna, established as a military fortress-colony to check the encroachments of Bedouin marauders, the practice of building well-drained toilets adjoining public buildings was customary in town planning.[13]

Looking back to the ideas presented by Cato, Celsus and Columella makes it clear that the Romans had no concept of a public hospital to care for the sick. The Roman in the non-military world of the early Empire assumed that sick citizens were cared for in the traditional way. The Roman, as he took care of his household, provided what Celsus calls *ampla valetudinaria* for those who were ill or needed rest.[14] Medical aid was given, according to Celsus, in the master's household. The master supervised the work of the physicians he consulted.[15] Columella notes it was best to have *valetudinaria* available for slaves who needed a period of rest and recuperation.

For the origins of care for the sick in public institutions, one looks to the newly arrived Christianity. It seems that the early Christians remembered the words of their Master, 'I was sick, and

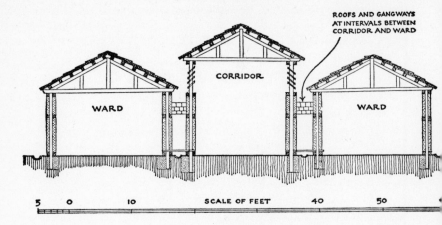

Figs 4, 5 Cross-section of the wards and corridors of the legionary hospital at Inchtuthil as restor the late Professor Sir Ian Richmond, based on the ground plan opposite. This is probably based the Roman aristocratic valetudinarium

ye visited me', and thought the care of the sick was a duty special to their own belief.[16] By AD 150, the Christians had the custom of collecting donations every Sunday for 'orphans, widows, those who are in want owing to sickness. . .'.[17] This sort of informal care was probably all that existed in the shape of 'public' care, and it was not widespread until the days of Julian. Eusebius is not aware of organized hospitals, but Julian makes special reference to them as he advises his priests to imitate the Christians at their best.[18] Thus the Romans, particularly in the West, continued the old tradition of household medicine for their immediate use, and until the Christian religion took hold of the crumbling Roman West, there were no true public hospitals.[19]

Many of the sanitary techniques in practice in the Roman *castra*, as seen in the military *valetudinaria* in the early Empire, were used in differing ways by Roman society in civilian answers to similar problems. Latrines, well-drained or with provision for a semi-sanitary maintenance, became commonplace among the houses of the wealthy in Rome and elsewhere in the Empire.[20] Baths, which formed an important part of many of the military centres in the

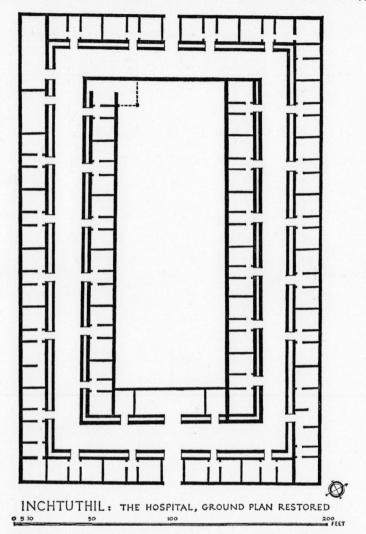

INCHTUTHIL: THE HOSPITAL, GROUND PLAN RESTORED

0 5 10   50   100   200
                                                        FEET

north, became a symbol of the Roman concern for the general welfare of the public at large. The imperial baths, both in the frontier areas and in the urban centres of the Empire, were justly famous, and their ruins are impressive and complex.[21] The Roman relaxed here, and even showed off his oratorical skill because the walls and the moisture of the baths gave resonance not attainable

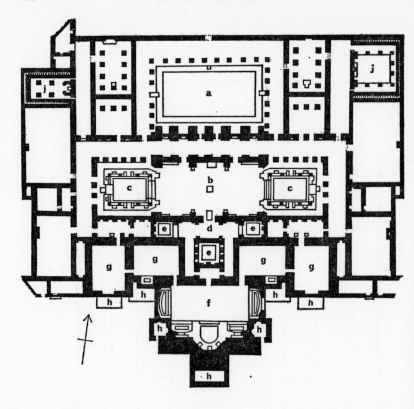

Fig. 6 Hadrian's Baths at Lepcis Magna (AD *126–7*) *show a mature and formal plan. The building included:* A *an open-air swimming bath;* B *frigidarium;* C *plunge baths;* D *tepidarium;* E *a large central and two smaller baths;* F *calidarium;* G *superheated rooms;* H *furnaces; and* J *latrines*

in the open air.[22] Within the structure of the baths, the Roman architect built adequate facilities for public waste disposal, and in light of their general reliability and majesty, one scholar has gone so far as to theorize upon the architectural planning and resultant efficiency as a conscious expression by the Romans of their power over the physical world.[23]

The Roman hygienic advance is well illustrated in the works of Varro and Columella. From a generalized hunch, Varro anticipated the germ theory of disease, but one cannot assume, as has been done, that the Romans did any more than speculate upon causes to explain the effects that they witnessed.[24] Lucretius and the Epicurean school—the 'live' universe—is in mind as Varro writes:

> Especial care should be taken, in locating the steading, to place it at the foot of a wooded hill, where there are broad pastures, and so as to be exposed to the most healthful winds that blow in the region. . . . Precautions must also be taken in the neighbourhood of swamps, both for the reasons given, and because there are bred certain minute creatures which cannot be seen by the eyes, which float through the air and enter the body through the mouth and the nose and there cause serious diseases.[25]

Then Varro continues the dialogue, with a typically Roman, practical, near-avaricious attitude, and the Roman answer to disease-causing areas.

> 'What can I do', asked Fundianus, 'to prevent disease if I should inherit a farm of that kind?' 'Even I can answer that question,' replied Agrius; 'sell it for the highest cash price; or if you can't sell it, abandon it.' Scrofa, however, replied: '. . . do not build in a hollow, but rather on elevated ground, as a well-ventilated place is more easily cleared if anything obnoxious is brought in. Furthermore, being exposed to the sun during the whole day, it is more wholesome, as any animalculae which are bred near by and brought in are either blown away or quickly die from the lack of humidity.[26]

Columella follows this pattern, with a sharply worded con-demnation of the lack of medical knowledge for problems of this kind.

> Nor, indeed, should there be a marshy area near to the build-ings, nor next to a public highway; for a marsh always emits noxious and poisonous vapours during the hot periods of the summer, and, at this time, gives birth to animals possessing

mischief-making stings, which fly to us in very thick swarms; thus, too, the swamp emits, from the mud and fermented dirt, poisonous pests in the form of water snakes and serpents which have been deprived of the moisture that they lived in during the winter; thus unknown diseases are often contracted, the causes of which even trained physicians cannot understand with any assurance.[27]

The Roman, as he sought to answer the vexing questions concerning the health of a farm and its location, found he could deal best with them in the terms well enunciated by Cato.[28] Avoidance of the problem was the solution, since the Roman could not combat diseases effectively, and malaria must have ravaged these areas from time to time, and made them even more impracticable for agriculture. Formal medicine had little impact in the Roman consideration of disease and its economic effects on the farm. Nevertheless, Roman practical acumen allowed a certain amount of experimental understanding of the problems involved, and Roman agriculture, sometimes patterned after Hellenistic precedents in the Empire, showed an achievement of living with disease. Hardiness of the individual was as important for the Roman farmer as it always has been in agricultural pursuits.[29]

In addition to indicating the physical expression of Roman efficiency in practical medical matters, archaeology has shown something of the Roman adaptability in regard to medical apparatus. Finds of medical instruments throughout the Roman Empire indicate that the art of surgery had progressed and proliferated. If any branches of medicine had true competence in the Empire, surgery—particularly the superficial, non-abdominal variety—is the most serviceable example. Surgery was important in the training of the conscientious physician, and both Celsus and Galen emphasize it although they came from divergent medical traditions.[30]

Technical competence in surgery became better as new shapes were devised for medical tools, and as new metals and alloys were found to provide sharper edges and cheaper equipment.[31] In the Empire, the doctor was supposedly the master of many branches

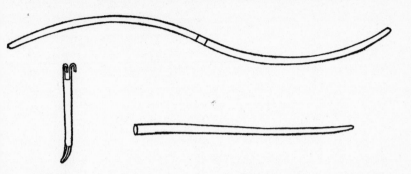

Figs 7–9 Above, *male catheter,* below, *female catheter* (see *Galen XIV, 787; Paul VI, 19, and Celsus VII, 26*). *The male catheter was probably useful in treatment of what modern medicine labels as cancer of the prostrate gland as well as to empty the bladder in cases of sphincter malfunction. Left, an arrow scoop (see Celsus VII, 5). Our reconstruction is highly conjectural based upon Celsus' description, which may show handbook consultation rather than field experience (see Plate 18)*

of medical knowledge, including what passed for pharmacology. The legions experienced the services of physician-drug pounders, and their craft was passed along for many generations. Technical specialities—or at least what the Romans distinguished among the drug dealers—appeared and received their share of jibes. If the physician pursued his studies carefully, he emerged with some knowledge of drugs, some understanding of medical tools, and a little understanding of internal anatomy. His experience in surgery gave him a good knowledge of superficial anatomy, particularly musculature of the arms and legs.[32] Surgery was highly refined as long as the patient had courage and the doctor had good tools and experience, and the head and the abdomen were not involved. A cursory reading of Celsus' summary of surgical techniques as they existed in the first century shows sense and firm purpose, as well as a reasonably sure knowledge of human anatomy.

The best illustration of sophisticated Roman surgical tools is Milne's collection of plates and commentary. Improvement by the Romans on earlier patterns, particularly in military surgical tools, is apparent from numerous examples. Celsus, in describing

what Milne calls an 'arrow scoop', speaks of the instrument as
sometimes being '. . . made of iron', as the Greeks used it, but
then Celsus inserts that it can be made 'even from bronze'.[33] The
description of the arrow scoop is confusing, and the diagram is
based upon what Milne pictures it to be.[34] Galen suggests Roman
sophistication with medical utensils in his description of a catheter.[35] Other references to the catheter and archaeological finds
make it possible to have a clear idea of what the Roman physician
used as he speaks of this instrument. Galen and later references
describe bone forceps, as well as catheters, and Milne describes the
forceps as follows:

> It is formed of two crossed branches moving on a pivot. The
> handles are square, the jaws are curved, and have across the
> inside of them parallel grooves which oppose each other
> accurately. It is classified . . . as an instrument for crushing
> calculus of the bladder.[36]

Fortunately for patients in the Roman Empire, the Museum of
Naples Catalogue's description probably was inaccurate, and such
an operation was performed with a chisel of fine dimensions.[37]

In smaller instruments, a refinement of medical technique and
the skill of manufacture are evident. Galen, Celsus, Scribonius
Largus, and Marcellus Empiricus mention the strigil as often used
to get into small openings.[38] Galen says, 'After having heated the
fat of a squirrel in a strigil, insert it into the auditory canal.'[39]

Milne shows that the Roman world had an abundance of well-
made surgical tools, and offers proof that often they were used
with great skill.[40] Archaeological remains of what appear to be
surgeons' shops are common enough to indicate physicians
specialized in surgery.[41] Particularly famous is the so-called House
of the Surgeon at Pompeii, where most of the surgical tools
housed in the Museum at Naples were found. It has been suggested
that the over-all plan of the House of the Surgeon indicates an
established practice, with a waiting room, an operating room, and
a certain amount of planning for sanitary drainage.[42] It appears,
however, that one is dealing with a summer resort, and not with

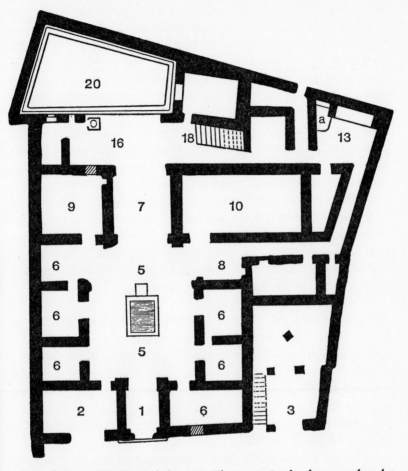

Fig. 10 'House of the Surgeon', Pompeii. *The assumption has been prevalent that because surgical tools were found in this house it warranted the designation given. The normal booths found on the front of the house would rather suggest an iron-monger's shop. 1 Entrance; 2, 3 Shops; 5 Atrium; 6 Private rooms; 7 Tablinum; 8 Ante-room; 9, 10 Dining rooms; 13 Kitchen (a, hearth); 16 Portico; 18 Stairs to rooms over the rear of the house; 20 Garden*

one of the centres of medical practice in the Empire. Conclusions drawn from the evidence at Pompeii may be true for a country town, but not generally true for the Empire as a whole.

As far as dissection is concerned, Milne and the medical sources make reference to it often enough, and the tools used show the usual sophistication of concept and production. If we are to trust the medical sources themselves, much of the Roman physician's mental energy was spent in speculation, and in his rejection or acceptance of a predetermined theoretical base for his medical activity. Although the tools existed for experimental dissection, it seems that the Roman doctor, by and large, learned his anatomy from practical experience, as did the *medicus* associated with the legion. The physician who entered his practice with a solid knowledge of anatomy was an exception, as Galen indicates from some of the obvious blunders of his colleagues.[43] Thus even with the sophistication in surgical instruments, we cannot conclude that the surgeon's skill matched the process which produced the tools he possessed. The intangible factor of collaborative technology moving with an age tuned to experimental thought must be considered as we view the Roman physician, and the lack of the first restrained a 'scientific' use of the technically well manufactured surgical utensils available in the Empire.

Galen remarks that the best quality of steel for the making of surgical tools came from Noricum.[44] In the case of a knife or a scalpel, the instrument sought was one not easily blunted, chipped, or bent.[45] In the making of such tools, the Roman founders searched for the finest ores, containing at least 75 per cent iron, and then working with a charcoal fuel, nearly pure carbon, they produced a fine quality of steel in limited amounts as easily as they could iron.[46]

Although high-quality steel tools could be made, the great majority of the surgical tools produced in the Roman world were made of bronze. Traditionally, the Hippocratic schools advised using only bronze for such instruments.[47] This had a practical rationale for the manufacture of the tools. Copper ore was more easily obtained and worked than iron, and the market was supplied with bronze surgical tools far less expensive than the steel ones. Most physicians took the advice of Hippocrates seriously and used bronze tools.[48] Other metals were used from time to time according to the need. Drugs were stored in copper bowls, and pure copper was occasionally used to make surgical tools.[49] Gold had varied uses: Hippocrates bound the teeth together in a jaw fracture with gold wire;[50] one later physician recommends use of a gold cautery to stop bleeding from the throat; tin vessels and boxes were used for the storage of certain drugs.[51] Milne describes a number of instances where silver was used in the manufacture of medical spoons, probes, drug boxes, bleeding cups, ligulae and styli for use in minor surgery, catheters, and even uterine syringes.[52] Bone was used to make ligulae and knives employed in the preparation of drugs.[53] Ivory was used to make a pestle found in a surgeon's outfit from Cologne.[54] Horn made good larger syringes.[55] The profusion of surgical tools from the Roman Empire is impressive, and indicates that the Roman understood the practical medical problems involved.

Turning from the technical and surgical accomplishments of the Empire to the general Roman concepts of public hygiene and sanitation, we find the Romans dealing with problems in a manner that still excites admiration. The Romans were sometimes squeamish in their formal references to such matters as urination and defecation, yet they managed to solve the problems of public waste disposal and sanitary water supply and use with consummate skill and forethought.[56] Even the early Republic witnessed the draining of the central marsh and the lowering of the ground water level of the Forum by the building of the Cloaca Maxima.[57] The Roman was motivated by a sense of propriety in the building of this great sewage system, and the description given by Pliny clarifies the sense of a standard attitude toward sanitation.[58] Although Pliny spends more time on the healing qualities of various springs around the Empire than he does on the sanitation systems themselves, he makes amply clear that the Roman sought clean water because it was necessary for good health.[59] Seneca bubbles over with pride about the Roman Empire, which had produced the finest baths and the best public sanitation system in the world:

Who would not think himself poor, indeed, if he bathed in a room that did not have walls that shine with the fiery brilliance of fine jewels? If the marble from Egypt were not

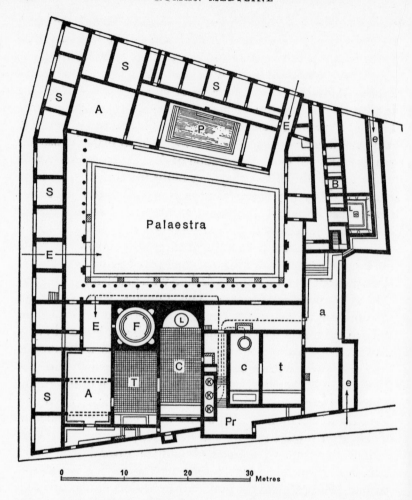

Fig. 11 *Stabian Baths, Pompeii.* S *Shops;* B *Private Baths;* A–T *Men's Bath* E; *Entrances;* A *Apodyteria;* F *Frigidarium;* T *Tepidarium;* C *Caldarium;* K *Kettles in furnace room;* P *Piscina;* L *Latrine;* Pr *Praefurnium. Lower case letters indicate areas reserved for women*

interspersed with the marble of Numidia, and were not panelled with mosaics? If the ceiling were not lined with crystal? If the clear water did not flow from silver faucets? And yet, I speak merely of the baths of the people.[60]

The Romans took for granted the superb system of baths, sewage and aqueducts, and came to expect this sort of public facility as a matter of course in the everyday life of the Empire.[61]

Vitruvius, as a practising architect in the milieu of the Roman Empire, shows through his writing how important sanitary planning was for public buildings. He was well aware of the medical implications of his work, and was influenced by the Pneumatic medical sect.[62] As a guidebook of architectural principles, *On Architecture* reflects much that is Hellenistic, but reveals the Roman practical tone noted in Cato, Varro, and Columella. The Roman utilitarian mind is at work, and Vitruvius' views on health show the careful observation of nature that one sees in Celsus and Columella.

The Site of a City.

For fortified towns the following principles are to be observed. First comes the choice of a very healthy site. Such a site will be high, neither misty nor frosty, and in a climate neither hot nor cold, but temperate; further, without marshes in the neighbourhood. For when the morning breezes blow towards the town at sunrise, if they bring with them mists from the marshes and, mingled with the mist, the poisonous breath of the creatures of the marshes, to be wafted into the bodies of the inhabitants, they will make the site unhealthy. . . . If one wishes a more accurate understanding of all this, he need only consider and observe the natures of birds, fishes, and land animals, and he thus will come to reflect upon distinctions of temperament.

Vitruvius also speaks of water supply as most important for the maintenance of good health, both publicly and privately:

. . . we must take great care and pains in searching for springs and selecting them, keeping in view the health of mankind. . . . If springs run free and open, inspect and observe the physique of the people who dwell in the vicinity before beginning to conduct the water, and if their frames are strong, their complexions fresh, legs sound, and eyes clear,

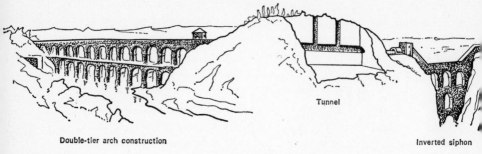

Double-tier arch construction Tunnel Inverted siphon

Fig. 12 A hypothetical aqueduct, according to Vitruvius and Frontinus, incorporating engineering problems the Romans faced in transporting water over long distances (after Hadas)

> the springs deserve complete approval. . . . If such water is
> boiled in a bronze cauldron . . . without sand or mud being
> found at the bottom of the cauldron, that water will have
> proved its excellence.[63]

Running water is Vitruvius' usual choice, and although the Roman
was not aware of ground water contamination, both Vitruvius
and Frontinus sought water supplies from upland areas where
such considerations would not apply.[64] It is fitting tribute to the
Roman architectural and sanitary ability that some of the aqueducts built in the Empire are still in use for the city of Rome.[65]

The aqueducts of Rome and her Empire were one of the major
glories of the classical world, and their stateliness and beauty as
some of them marched over the open countryside evoked admiration; they were true triumphs of Roman sanitary engineering.
Nine of the eleven aqueducts of ancient Rome are described in
Frontinus' *Aqueducts*. Frontinus had been a soldier who had
become Praetor of the City of Rome, Augur, three times Consul
(75, 98, 100), governor of Britain (76–78), and was appointed
water commissioner (*Curator aquarum*) in 97. The Roman practical
genius shows its best side in the work of Frontinus, who approached his massive job with balance and a sense of the duty he

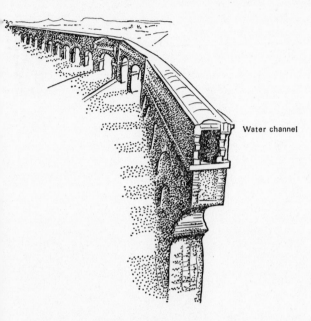

Water channel

had for the health of Rome. He recognized the sanitary aspects of his position, and states bluntly, 'my office . . . concerns not only the usefulness of such a system, but also the very health and safety of Rome. . . .'[66] Frontinus' conscientiousness is further reflected as he expresses his concepts of public health:

> One can observe the effect of this care . . . on the queen and empress of the world, and it can be observed even more in the improved health of Rome because of the greater number of reservoirs, works, fountains, and water basins. . . . the appearance of Rome is cleaner and changed, and the causes of the unhealthy atmosphere, that gave Rome so bad a name among the ancients, are now removed.[67]

Frontinus hints that the Roman may be aware of the advantages of having water coming into the city which has run over rocks and small stones, and he describes a kind of filter box (*piscina*) through which water runs among some sand.[68]

As Frontinus describes the aqueducts, the modern reader is impressed with the efficiency of their construction and their operation. The Romans reared the majestic cross-valley aqueducts solely for economic and structural reasons. Lead piping underground was weak, bronze was far too expensive, and the casting of large pipes which could resist the tremendous pressures involved was beyond Roman technology. Inverted siphons were used, showing that the Romans were aware that water seeks its own level, and the inverted siphonage was often used to good advantage for supplying fountains in the upper levels of the more expansive houses.[69]

The Roman technical and hygienic achievement, seen in its proper perspective, clearly outweighs the purely medical advances. Celsus delineates the Roman concept of health in similar ways as do Vitruvius and Frontinus: it was far more important to maintain health than it was to depend upon the medical practice of the day, be it Greek or Roman. The generalized attitude was reflected in the magnificent structures which symbolized Roman solutions to the questions of public health and its maintenance, and the concept forms a continuum with the ancient idea that health was an individual concern in the framework of the great household.

In a later time, Vegetius summarized the attitude as it had emerged from an earlier Roman Empire. The tone is that of Varro, Celsus, Columella, and Cato, and the Roman practical common sense is dominant, rather than a dependence upon medicine as a separate discipline.

> I will now give some indications as to how the health of the army is to be preserved and maintained, in relation to locations of the camps, purity of water, temperature, medicine, and exercise. In regard to spots to place a camp, soldiers must not remain for too long near the locations of unhealthy marshes. . . . They ought not to begin their march too late in the day, lest they contract disease due to the sun's heat or the fatigue that would result from the journey. . . . the soldier who must endure cold without proper clothing is not in a state to have good health or to march . . . nor must he use

swamp waters for drinking purposes. . . . those who are most knowledgeable in military matters are of the opinion that daily exercise contributes far greater health to the soldiers than do the physicians. . . . If a number of soldiers are allowed to stay in one locale too long in the summer or the autumn, they suffer from corruption of the water supply, and are rendered miserable by the smell of their own excrement, and the very air is made unhealthy . . . and grave disease afflicts them. . . . this has to be corrected . . . by moving to another camp-site.[70]

CHAPTER VII

THE PUBLIC ESTIMATE OF ROMAN MEDICINE

AQUEDUCTS AND BATHS provided the population of the Roman Empire with health-promoting structures, symbolic of the concern the Roman Imperial government had for its peoples. For the hygienic accomplishments, our evidence is relatively clear, but for individual reaction to medical practice in the daily run of life, we see only fragments of the broad social picture. Most of what we know comes from the literature of the Roman upper classes, but even here many medical problems in all classes of Roman society are revealed with some clarity.

Roman literature contains much which tells us about the reactions of individuals to medicine and doctors in the Empire. One notes a surprising uniformity in Latin sources. They show a combination of traditional concepts of health with a scepticism of practising Greek physicians. The educated public at large exhibits a rational balance concerning medicine and its effectiveness, and this contrasts with the medical sources, which suffer from attempts at self-justification.

Suggestions that the poet Horace was a good friend of Celsus[1] rest on tenuous evidence. The poet's opinion of doctors in his day was ambivalent, and he recognized several sorts of physicians. The poorer classes were cared for by *pharmocopolae* who dispensed drugs.[2] The poor could rely upon the time-tested protection of the Roman deities, as we noted in Cato.

When Diana hears the call, given three times a day by a young woman in the pangs of childbirth, she snatches them from death.[3]

Ignorant doctors were common, and a badly veiled sarcasm touches his verse as Horace speaks of them.

> Where is the man
> Who ventures to administer a draught
> Without due training in the doctor's craft?
> Doctors prescribe who understand the rules
> And only workmen handle workmen's tools.[4]

Horace gives credit to good physicians, but again his verse shows they were far rarer than the incompetent. The Roman had to ponder carefully before committing himself to the care of one of the resident medical practitioners.

> The false caution of the foolish will hide ulcers in preference
> to having them cured.[5]

Probably quacks of both Greek and Latin origins abounded in Rome, but Greeks figure in our sources with great regularity while others acquire the characteristics of Hellenistic doctors. Horace was puzzled by the differences between the Hellenistic and Roman outlooks on health,[6] but managed a smooth synthesis of both cultures in his work.[7] None the less he rejected the greedy attitudes of his Empire in Roman bluntness and Hellenistic theory, and sometimes he passed his quandary off in a few gloomy references as he returned to his craft of poetry.[8]

Doctors had the reputation of being privy to plots involving poison, and Horace warns his reader not to trust the medical practitioner.[9] Martial's attitude is common.

> Oft with thy wife does the physician lie,
> Thou knowing, Charidem, and standing by.
> I see that thou wilt not of a fever die.[10]

In apparent contrast, Seneca offers praise for the physician, but his statements are vague and give interesting depictions of the relation between the doctor and his patients in the Empire. At one point, Seneca writes, 'you pay a doctor for something beyond value, life and excellent health . . .'[11] But Seneca has something other than our 'professional' in mind. The physician becomes a friend if he is good at what he does,[12] and Seneca's praise is reserved for the unique sort of doctor-compatriot (slave or otherwise) and not for the physician who performs his job and receives his fees.[13] The reference reminds one of the ambiguous tone of Horace, but Seneca speaks in the role of the powerful aristocrat who 'commands' physicians[14] and who values them for their intellect and compassion.

The imperial household provides a striking example of the attitude the educated Roman had towards the Greek physician. The imperial government officially encouraged the settlement of Greek doctors and teachers in Rome, but our sources mention these gentlemen with reservations.[15] Few Romans took the trouble to learn the methods of the Greek physician, and the craft associated with the imperial house was confined to Greeks and those of Greek extraction.[16] The Emperor Claudius revealed the Roman interest in medicine. Schooled as a youth by the historian Livy, Claudius as Emperor exhibited his interest in history, and was fascinated by influences from the Hellenistic east. Two examples of purported medicine from the east captivated him.

Claudius' personal physician was Xenophon of Cos and, on his behalf, Claudius proposed the island be relieved of taxation. In the speech in part recorded by Tacitus, Claudius retailed an obviously fictional pedigree for Xenophon, going back to Aesculapius, the founder of medicine.[17] Tacitus' use of the opportunity to ridicule medicine has given us a garbled version of the episode. With his best irony, Tacitus notes how the faithful physician, with the aid of Agrippina, helped Claudius to his end.[18] The second instance showing this interest by Claudius is a letter from Thessalus of Tralles. Claudius was addressed, and the letter considers the virtue of medicinal plants in relation to the signs of the zodiac.[19] The whole essay is steeped in Near Eastern superstition, proving the great difficulty the Roman had in separating medicine from folklore as it emerged from the Hellenistic east.[20]

The Roman patient became increasingly disillusioned with the Greek physician. The attitude became more caustic. Another passage from Tacitus brings the fashionable sarcasm clearly to the attention of his readers, as well as the contrast between Greek and

Roman views of medicine. While the Emperor Vespasian was at Alexandria, he was asked to try his ability at healing.[21] Serapis advised two sufferers to ask Vespasian for a cure.[22] Their request perplexed Vespasian and he turned to the city physicians for a diagnosis. Tacitus renders their pompous reply in professionally artificial words. The physicians thought it wise to conduct the experiment as it 'perhaps was the will of the gods . . . if a cure were effected, the credit would go to the ruler.'[23] If it did not succeed, then ridicule would fall on the poor cripples. Tacitus may reflect what most of his class felt about Hellenistic physicians.

Evidence for public mistrust of the physicians is plentiful, including a large number of epigrams from the *Greek Anthology*.

The physician Marcus laid his hand yesterday on the stone Zeus, and though he is of stone and Zeus, he is to be buried today.[24]

Phidon did not purge me with a clyster or even feel me, but feeling feverish I remembered his name and died.[25]

Alexis the physician purged by a clyster five patients at one time, and five others by drugs; he visited five, and again he rubbed five with ointment. And for all there was one night, one medicine, one coffin-maker, one tomb, one Hades, one lamentation.[26]

Socles, promising to set Diodorus' crooked back straight, piled three solid stones, each four feet square, on the hunch-back's spine. He was crushed and died, but he became straighter than a ruler.[27]

These epitaphs are probably nothing more than personal bitterness at the individual physicians concerned. Nevertheless, the large number of similar examples bears out the conclusion that the physician was feared, and consulted only in the last resort.

Quackery was rife on all levels of society. Our sources often note fraudulent drug dealers. The chicanery was so prevalent as to touch almost anybody who needed a salve for a bruise or burn.[28] The best drugs were shipped to the imperial house, where they commanded exorbitant prices.[29] Doctors carried drug lists with which they issued prescriptions but were often ignorant of the properties in the ingredients. The Roman viewed such matters as close to scandalous, but accepted it as a part of the usual conduct of the physician, who said he knew much, but was ignorant of even the simplest medical facts.[30]

> Some doctors charge the most excessive prices for the most worthless medicines and drugs, and others in the craft attempt to deal with and treat diseases they obviously do not understand. . . .[31]

Drug sellers came from many classes of society, and the physician was forced to deal with 'unmedical' individuals in order to procure his medicaments.

> . . . drugs make medicine clear to the user and to the doctor, and the physician must spare no effort to have a great knowledge of medical recipes, and he must consult persons who are not part of the medical craft. These often succeed where doctors fail.[32]

The stereotyped doctor was supposed to enter the sickroom, bleed the patient, lay on a plaster, and give an enema.[33] Doctors gave advice to cure everything (one remedy) from headaches to dislocated shoulders.[34] The quackery got so bad in some places that the good doctors asked their patients to be the best judge of the problems.[35] The patient took fraud for granted even in trivial matters of medical interest.

Loathsome materials were prescribed since the physicians thought these ingredients—centipedes, human faeces, and the like —carried greater power than ordinary drugs.[36] Galen does not think such drugs are always useful, but he lists them anyway, noting their popularity with his predecessors.[37] Drug dealers made their way over the whole of the Empire, and we possess clear evidence of a booming drug trade carried on in the name of curing those who bought the salves and soothing ointments.[38] Public mistrust for the drug dealer was widespread, if we are to believe Pliny, who tells us certain streets and locations where drugs were made became bywords for cheating and sloppy work.[39]

Doctors competed with one another for their patients, and physicians (and those who said they were doctors) employed lectures to impress city crowds. Sometimes it worked. Sometimes it did not.

> This sort of recitation . . . is a kind of spectacle or parade . . . like the exhibitions of the so-called physicians, who seat themselves conspicuously before us and give a detailed account of the union of joints, the combination and juxta-position of bones, and other topics of that sort, such as pores and respirations, and excretions. And the crowd is all agape with admiration and more enchanted than a swarm of children.[40]

Lucian has the travelling quack in mind as he writes, 'you are similar to the fake physicians who buy themselves silver cupping-glasses, lancets with gold handles, all encased in ivory. But they do not know how to use the tools when the time comes and make way for a proper doctor who produces a knife with a sharp edge, but which has a rusty handle. . . .'[41] Plutarch grumbles that it is 'sophistry to put on a show before onlookers as the doctors do in the theatres with the hope of attracting patients'.[42] Practitioners used all sorts of questionable methods to gain patients, ranging from escorting the prospective patient home to sharing dirty jokes with him. Galen notes these fellows were well-equipped with fine clothes and fancy medical utensils, but lacked medical theory. Such charlatans did good work only by lucky chances and even then they arrived at their conclusions through false premises. They took little time to learn medicine, but proclaimed to their many followers that medicine could be learned quickly. The cities granted them the right to 'waste time' since these doctors pleased the throng looking for expensive rings, silver medical tools, and a large claque of followers as criteria for medical success. The man of judgement turned away from the common-place doctor, and listened to the medicine Galen taught, which was 'different from all these'.[43]

Galen heaps contempt on the physician who employed flattery in his quest for patients. The lower-class doctor recalled each name of the rich and powerful as he passed them on the street. He acted as the 'bodyguard of the mealtimes', as a common slave would do, and escorted his patient home at the end of the day, taking care that his fawning and flattery were not lost upon the rich man he was going to cheat. Galen gives the impression these doctors were a part of a great group of clients swarming around the influential men of Rome and the cities of the Empire, and who gained employment through blandishments.[44]

Public response to Hellenistic theories is vividly illustrated in the medicine practised in Roman Egypt. Here the native traditions maintained their strength in the face of Hellenism and the Roman rule, and it was only in the declining years of the Empire that Egypt became integrated into the Empire. By then the dry rot was apparent.

> Psasinus appeared before the praefect and said, 'I am a doctor by profession, and I have treated these same people who have assigned me a public burden,' and Eudaimon said, 'Perhaps you treated them incorrectly. If you are a doctor, practising mummification, tell me what is the solvent, and you will receive the immunity you claim.'[45]

The impact of Hellenistic medicine on the people of Egypt was not great, and other papyri attest that most turned to accepted methods and found little to attract them in Roman or Hellenistic medicine.[46]

Roman Gaul provides evidence elucidating common attitudes about medical care administered on the great country estates in the Empire. A will from Langres explicitly directs the relatives and servants of the deceased to cremate all of the equipment he had acquired for the purpose of 'hunting and fowling'. The list of materials includes 'lances, swords, knives, nets, snares . . . and all the medicines and tools which relate to that activity . . .'.[47] The preceding passages of the will suggest the normal Roman chapel and exedra with a statue of the deceased, as well as specific instructions on materials and stone for the memorial. The Gallic custom of cremation of the gentleman's dearest possessions was one of long standing,[48] yet the elaboration of the memorial shrine was common among the Roman aristocracy. The master of the house considered the medical instruments and ointments to be his, and ordered that they be destroyed with his hunting apparel. The Gallo-Roman will of the early second century bears proof of the aristocratic concepts Celsus illustrated for Rome in the first century.

Celsus lets us see something of the generalized Roman scepticism towards Hellenistic medicine, as he notes how chance can do more for a man than can medicine. 'Since fortune aids very much in the curing of diseases,' Celsus writes, 'consideration of diet and drugs', among other matters, can all at the same time be very helpful and of no use whatever. It is therefore a moot point 'whether health reappears because of medicine or a healthy body or simply good luck'.[49]

In one aspect, public response to Hellenistic theories yielded positive results. This is not to say the complex phenomenon making use of speculation, religion, magic, astrology, folk therapeutics, and the rest, did not often give positive and practical results, but to note that the results could not be predicted with reliability. In contrast the Romans used the medicine of their day with predictable results in applying methods of contraception.

Hellenistic medicine taught the methods and concepts of contraception. Use of contraceptives was limited in the Empire to those who commanded the services of a Greek physician, and may have had far-reaching consequences. Desire for small families produced abortion on a large scale, particularly among the Roman aristocrats. Family size among this class was controlled deliberately by contraceptives and other means.[50] The Roman government realized the danger to the state involved in contraception, and the well-known laws of Augustus were the first of many attempts to encourage large numbers of children among the ruling class.[51] Contraceptive techniques used by the Romans showed that Hellenistic and Roman medicine had found solutions for the problem of unwanted children, which had a long history in the Greek and Hellenistic world.[52]

The same general problems existed in the Empire as do today. Those who used the methods available were the better educated and more 'desirable' elements of Roman society, and those who did not (or would not) proved to be the poorer segments with no real hope of feeding the new mouths sufficiently.[53] Even though Roman girls married young (age fifteen or so was about average), and about half of their marriages lasted about eighteen years, the number of children in the upper classes continued to fall.[54] Complicating matters was the lack of an 'ideal' faithful husband, and prostitution was common, as it was throughout the history of classical antiquity.[55]

Although there were many illiterate doctors practising medicine in the Empire, there were something like established centres of medical education, gaining a physician respect if he had studied at one of them.[56] The tradition of some excellence reinforced the importance of the tenets of Hellenistic medicine in the Empire, especially among the upper classes. Doctors serving the wealthier Romans knew contraceptive information, a tradition extending back to Hippocrates and Aristotle. Dioscorides and Pliny record a confused version of the tradition. Clearly what the Romans thought of as contraception is not the same as our concept.[57] Soranus does make clear the distinction between contraception and abortion, but more often the methods are described similar to 'a contraceptive (atokion) such as pepper should be applied after coitus'.[58]

Public response to medicine was related to social rank. The physician of quality served the citizen rich enough to employ him. Physicians of lesser repute campaigned among the masses for patients, and they lacked true skill and learning. Having observed their performances, the rank and file rejected both the physician and his theoretical base, since the one served no purpose and the other was meaningless jargon. As time passed, even the upper classes became disappointed with physicians, and our evidence is sharp in its criticism and clear concerning the response to medicine by the Roman intellectual.

Even though some doctors treated philosophy as one of their provinces, many turned away from it to concentrate on medicine and offended their more educated patients. Plutarch's ideal physician was one 'worth many men put together' and he borrows Homer's phrase to describe him. Glaucus, the physician who was harsh and hostile towards his patients, refuses to value philosophy. To refute him, Plutarch discusses medicine as an elegant and distinct part of the liberal arts. Philosophers should not put borders between the substance of medicine and philosophy, but make it one area of concern in knowing the enjoyable and the necessary. He feels anger against the philosopher who takes no interest in medicine, and, as an intelligent man, will raise himself above those who throng to watch the public performances of physicians. The rest of the *Instruction* puts forth general rules of health which educated men know and observe, especially in diet and exercise. Plutarch admits acquaintance with medical terms and literature, but suggests they are pedantic and used only when one wishes to display a sort of esoteric learning to the sick, who cannot profit from wordiness. Rather Plutarch inquires into causes, and compares his health with the problems bringing on his friend's illness. He throws his remarks into the realm of comparison of man's spiritual worth and his bodily health, and moderation and restraint are keys to Plutarch's presentation of health.[59] Diseases of the body are evils detected by the pulse and an excess of bile, which fever and sudden pains confirm. Plutarch asserts that evils of the soul are more important, but escape notice.[60] Thus men who suffer from spiritual evils are unaware of their true natures, and their affliction is the worse.

Plutarch had read widely in the medical literature of his day and he feels he can judge matters of health and disease as competently as any of the physicians. Plutarch's philosophy of medicine does not impress us with a depth of learning comparable to Galen, but Plutarch had little faith in medicine as a separate branch of knowledge which could aid men in their problems. Some of his conclusions on the temperaments of individuals and their constitutions resemble Galen's writing,[61] but Plutarch uses these terms to reassert his conviction of the intelligent man's ability to understand on his own.[62] Plutarch is no invalid, nor does he brood on his health as would the true valetudinarian, but his self-taught command of the medical essentials gives clues to the usual educated attitude on medicine and its worth.

Plutarch's home-learned medicine and its implications for the educated class in the Roman Empire provide some explanation for the hypochondria expressed by Statius, Fronto, and Aelius Aristides. They had some knowledge of medicine, and apparently felt sickly enough at the time to write about their health problems, which each solved in his own way. Statius does not note the skill of physicians but the healing powers of Apollo and Aesculapius, and his friend Rutilius Gallicus recovers at home under the care of his family. Statius tosses in every allusion he can in describing the recovery of Gallicus, from references to Chiron's herbs, Pergamon's reputation, Epidaurus' healing sands, to medical skill aided by Arabic perfumes. Gallicus receives drugs and his recovery is as swift as Statius' allusions to Vergil and Horace can make it.[63] True valetudinarianism appears as Statius tells us about his problems, and his wife, patient and tender, nurses him back to a semblance of health.[64] In lamenting the death of his adopted son, Statius mentions the ambiguity of medicine, and its greater use for his affliction—sorrow—than for the health of his dead son.[65]

Fronto, the esteemed tutor of the young Marcus Aurelius, was a bedevilled hypochondriac. He, too, displays a knowledge of medicine, and sees grave problems in himself. Pains in the elbow, knee, neck, and throughout his body plague Fronto, who discreetly moans to his royal pupil.[66] Then he is struck by pains in his groin, back, shoulders, and neck again, which send Fronto back to renew his vows before the Lares and Penates.[67] He tries drinking from health-giving springs, which helps for a while, but new attacks come which take away Fronto's voice, and even his consciousness—the physicians had given him up—but he gets better in three days with the help of the gods.[68] Then Fronto scrapes his knee, and somehow this leads back to his pains in the foot, stomach cramps, and the like, for which the doctors recommend a bath.[69] Next come a sore throat, more knee pains, a crippled hand, a nasty cough, which prevents Fronto from writing.[70] When Verus fell ill, Fronto tells us of the 'drastic bloodletting' which 'freed him from the danger of possible illness', and then Fronto 'made prayers at every hearth, altar, sacred grove, and consecrated tree'.[71] Meanwhile Fronto still has problems of his own. His limbs

24, 25 Private and public Roman lavatories at Ostia. Sanitary arrangements were far superior in the public lavatories where running water continually flushed below the marble seats. There is no evidence that the public facilities provided segregated the sexes. The modern idea of privacy was not held in Roman times as numerous examples of multiple seating public lavatories, as seen *below*, show.

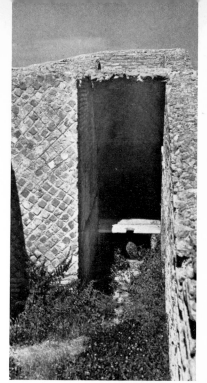

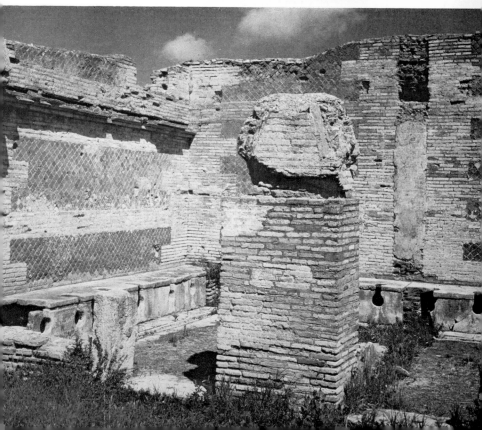

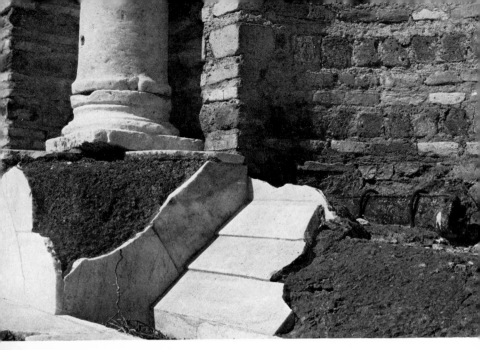

26, 27 Frontinus was much concerned with piped water through conduits such as that *above*, a lead pipe *in situ* at Ostia in the House of Amor and Psyche. *Below*, an excellent example of a two-seater lavatory at Timgad with decorative dolphin armrests. Apparently provision was made for the collection of the urine, used in cleaning by fullers.

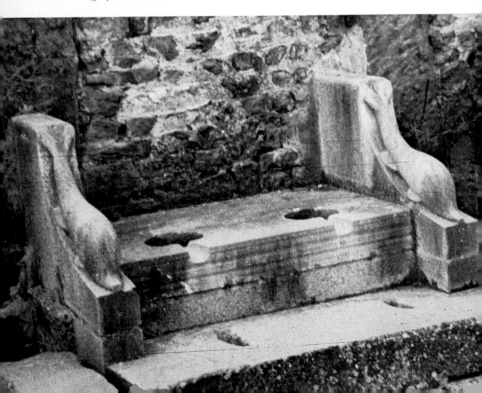

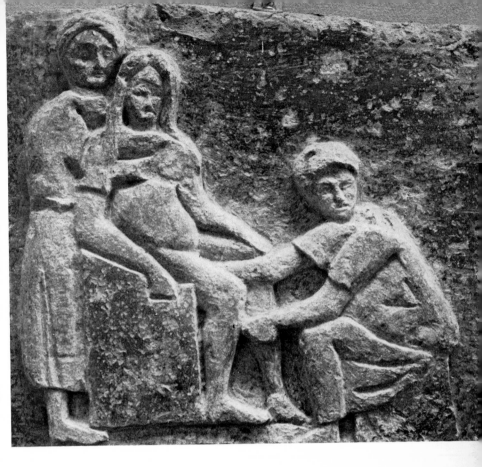

28, 29 Two medical reliefs from Ostia. *Above*, the midwife (as described by Soranus) performing a delivery whilst her colleague holds the patient who is seated in an 'obstetrical chair' grasping the special handles provided. *Below*, a surgeon, left, is performing what is probably a light blood-letting on the right leg of the patient. He uses a lancet and there is a bowl below for collecting the blood. Ostia Museum.

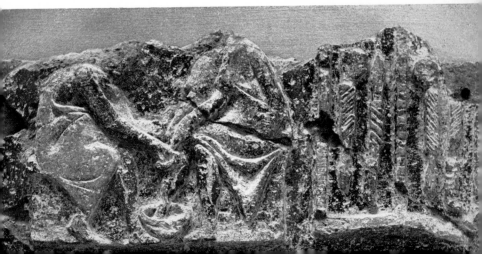

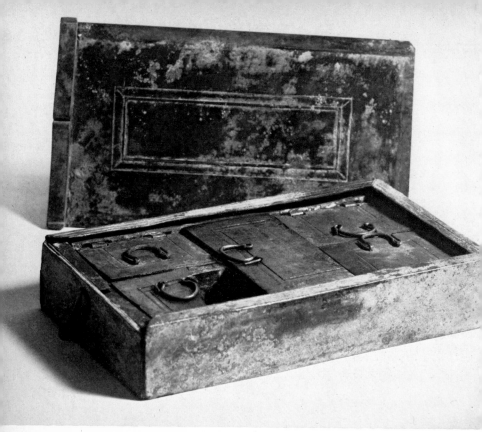

30 A Roman metal box divided into five compartments, possibly for carrying unguents or powders for medicinal use. Probably from Asia Minor. British Museum.

31 Wall painting from the House of the Vetii, Pompeii; one of a series showing amorini at work. Here they are probably preparing aphrodisiacs of various descriptions. Most likely the process illustrated is very similar to the actual preparation of drugs for public consumption (*cf.* Pliny XXXIV, 22-30). Naples Museum.

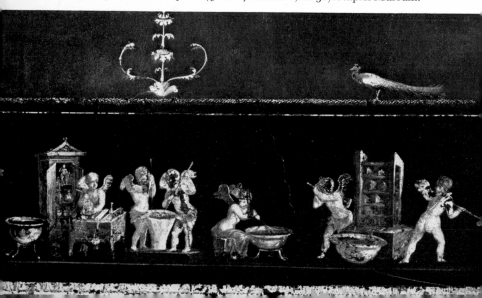

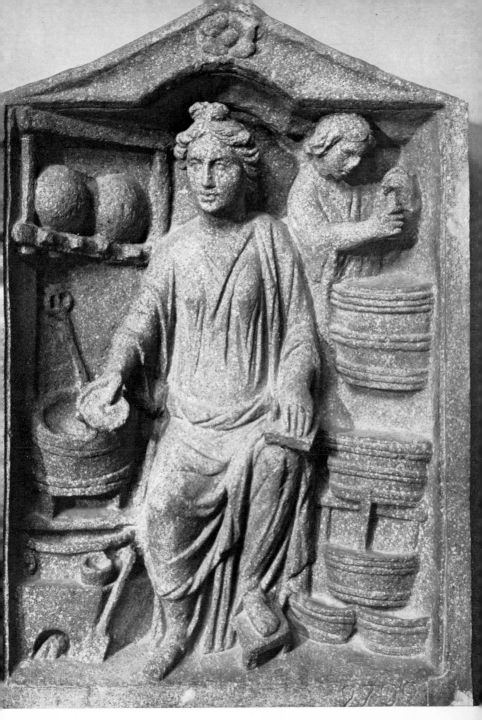

32 Relief showing soap and salve making. An assistant apparently grinds ingredients using a mortar and pestle. The products were simmered in a cauldron over a furnace, left, and stored in the vats, right. Epinal Museum.

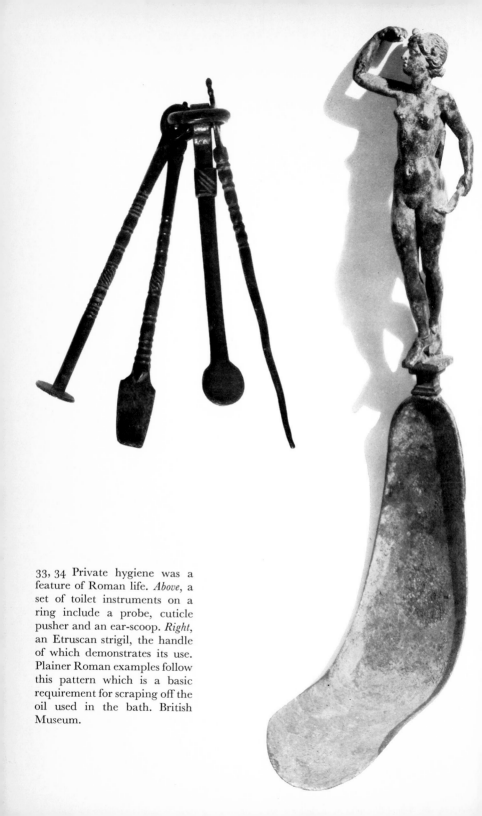

33, 34 Private hygiene was a feature of Roman life. *Above*, a set of toilet instruments on a ring include a probe, cuticle pusher and an ear-scoop. *Right*, an Etruscan strigil, the handle of which demonstrates its use. Plainer Roman examples follow this pattern which is a basic requirement for scraping off the oil used in the bath. British Museum.

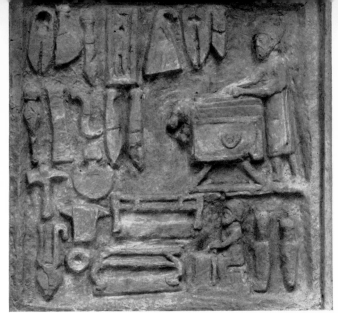

35, 36 Roman surgical tools were made by a blacksmith as the relief, *above*, from Ostia shows. Among the representations of his products we see surgical shears (top left), scalpels and probes interspaced amongst the expected hammers, tongs and hooks. *Below*, a more stylized representation of surgical instruments which includes scalpels, surgical tongs, a probe, cupping vessels, a syringe and what is probably an instrument case. Ostia and Lateran Museums.

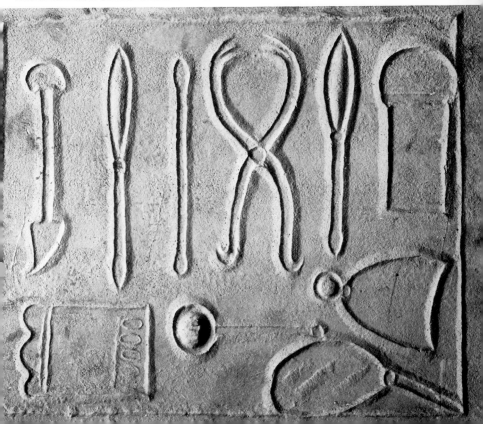

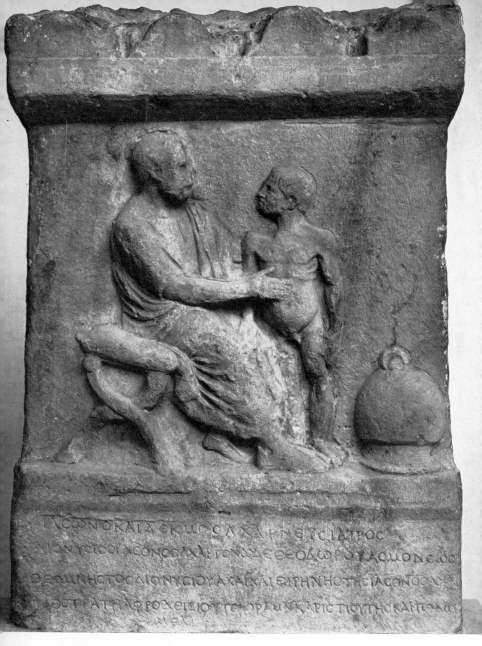

ΓΙ ΑΣ ΩΝ Ο ΚΑΙ ΔΕ ΚΜ ... Σ Α ΧΑ ... ΡΝ ΕΤΣ ΙΑΤΡΟΣ
ΔΙΟΝΥΣΙΟΟΙ ΑΣ ΩΝΟΣ Α ΧΑ ΓΟΝΟ Δ ΕΘΕΟΔΩΡΟΥ ΑΟΜΟΝ Ε ΙΟΟ
Ο ... ΟΔ Μ Η Σ ΤΟΣ ΔΙΟΝΥ Σ ΙΟΥ Α ΧΑ ΙΝΑΙ ΕΙΡΗΝΗ Σ ΤΗ Σ ΙΑΣ ΩΝΟΣ Α ...
... ΟΣ ΓΙ Α ΤΗ Α ΦΡΟΔ ΕΙΣ ΙΟΥ ΤΟ Π ... ΡΑ ... ΝΚΑΡΙΣ ΤΙ ΟΥ ΤΗ Σ ΚΑ ΡΠΟ Δ ...
... ΝΟΥ

37 The tombstone of Jason, an Athenian physician of the early second century AD. He is seen palpating the abdomen of a young boy who is probably suffering from the effects of malnutrition. To the right is a stylized and enlarged cupping vessel, suggesting that Jason may have specialized in bleeding methods using these vessels (*see* Plate 38). British Museum.

are subject to intense pain, as are his neck and groin.[72] Along the way, he makes rather witty fun of all the names known for his maladies,[73] but finds they are of little use. His long-time illnesses stay with him, even though he almost dreams himself into a cure for his rheumatism.[74]

The most eloquent valetudinarian of antiquity was Aelius Aristides. Born into the landed gentry of Asia Minor, he received the best education which the second century could offer.[75] One of his tutors was the Athenian Tiberius Claudius Atticus Herodes, the teacher of Marcus Aurelius in Greek oratory. Aristides became a master in his twenties of the best Attic style and was well acquainted with the great literature of the classical world and had travelled over much of the Roman Empire. When he was twenty-six, he went to Rome and gained an audience at the imperial court. Public affairs and oratory beckoned him into a great career and Aristides was set to become rich and famous. But he was laid low by a long series of diseases and maladies which made him an invalid for a dozen years and altered his personality for good.

His troubles varied in their intensity and time, but all bring forth a torrent of brooding by Aristides about himself, his career so rudely demolished, and particularly about Asclepius, who provides solace rather than a cure.[76] He tells us how he has been encouraged by his friends to put his experience down, but that it seemed impossible, as it would be similar to swimming under-water through each ocean and then telling how many waves he saw.[77] None the less, he is determined to persist in his task although every day had a tale of its own, as well as every night. Since sleep was rare during his sickliness, he feels he can obey the 'will of the god' as he might a doctor, and record what he remembers.[78] Dodds calls Aristides' illnesses 'of the psychosomatic type',[79] but the orator's feeling for his maladies is too real to be ignored. Symptoms bubble forth on almost every page, and modern classification recognizes acute bronchial asthma, hyper-tension, various shades of headaches, insomnia, and nasty gastric and intestinal disturbances.[80] Less clear are symptoms probably related to urinary calculi, pulmonary tuberculosis, prostatitis, typhoid fever, and perennial rhinitis.[81] Aristides suffers terribly from something that has many of the marks of tetanus and even undergoes a full-fledged convulsion which confuses rather than aids modern classification.[82] The sum of Aristides' illnesses is a hodge-podge of symptoms, seemingly borrowed from a number of diseases. As Dodds remarks, Aristides is a fit subject for a professional psychologist.[83]

Aristides has numerous contacts with physicians in his years of travail. When his tumour began to grow, the doctors prescribed caustic drugs or surgery, but the god advised the sufferer to bear it out. Aristides did for four months. Finally the god prescribed a particular sort of salty salve which caused the tumour to disappear. The doctors were amazed, and even dumbfounded when the god ordered Aristides to smear an egg on the loose fold of skin left from the tumour. The cure was so complete that the physicians could not discern where the tumour had been.[84] Doctors refused to give Aristides enemas when they saw how thin he was, but he insisted.[85] His good friend Zosimus was skilled in medicine, but died since he was sceptical of Aristides' medical dream-prophecies.[86]

Aristides enjoys confusing doctors, 'who were completely perplexed not only in how to aid me, but also in recognizing what it was that I had'.[87] Another doctor, Heracleon, gave a gloomy prognosis of spinal curvature for Aristides, which he cheerfully disregards in favour of the god's order to go and take a swim in an icy river (it was winter).[88] Then Aristides launches into a confused analysis of his bodily heats and coolness, wetness and aridity, concluding that his 'long-lasting body heat brought power to his whole body'. He gets satisfaction from telling us of how he jumped naked into the river and swam around, splashing happily for a long time, and received the applause of the gathered throng when he finally came out of the river. They, of course, shouted, 'Great is Asclepius!'[89]

Another doctor appears at the request of Aristides. He tells Theodotus, the physician, about his dreams, but all Theodotus would reply was something about how he feared for Aristides' condition in winter. The dreams, of course, were divine.[90] Later Aristides recovers from plague by a self-prescribed enema of

Attic honey and a meal of goose liver and sausage.[91] Bloodletting was so common for Aristides as to make one marvel that he survived at all. The usual incision was made at the elbow, but Aristides (following directions from a dream) has blood drawn from his forehead, just as Sedatius, a Roman senator, was being treated.[92] Once in a while, in his writing, Aristides flips back to the beginnings of his illness, and tells us of what the doctors did, from purging him with cucumber juice to making an incision from the chest to the bladder for the application of cupping instruments.[93] Doctors accompanied by gymnastic trainers did not help either.[94] While in Pergamon, Aristides was visited by the philosopher-physician, Satyrus. Satyrus was appalled by the great bloodletting, recommended that Aristides stop, and gave him a light ointment for his abdomen. Aristides complains that it was too cold to the touch, and thereupon he developed an awful cough and chest cold.

Aristides represents an intellectual response to medicine which borders upon the religious acceptance of Asclepian temple-medicine. Yet he shows excellent acquaintance with medical literature and doctors in his society, and rather than simply relegating him as a 'brainsick noodle with a religious sentiment both genuine and refined',[95] we should note the links with other reactions to medicine. Statius and Fronto fume about their illnesses, too, and treat themselves as best they can. They turn to home care and sacrifice to the traditional gods, as does Aristides. Physicians of all varieties hover in the shadows of all the valetudinarian accounts, suggesting, prescribing, demanding, offering philosophical reasoning and labels, but rarely curing. Even Satyrus, the best of the physicians that Aristides encounters, cannot give our megalomaniac hypochondriac what he needs. The other physicians are next to useless, giving advice when Aristides wants assurance. Of course, the modern reader may be justifiably suspicious of the motley presentation of what appear to be symptomatical inventions, but this is not the real importance of Aristides' long-winded description of himself. Dodds correctly sees Aristides as an example of the intellectual who finds a faith that fits his day. Galen admits dreams can help save lives,[96] but he puts his statement in terms of medical treatment which Aristides continually denies. 'Daylight reality was ceasing to be trusted',[97] fits the unrewarded bustle of Statius and Fronto, the fuzzy wordiness of the kind-hearted Plutarch, and Aristides, the hypochondriac looking for a companion larger than life. The intellectuality of Galen fails to pierce a growing gloom of an age gradually turning from the rational answers posed by the Greek heritage of questioning to the mystical, all-encompassing solutions of religion.

The Romans viewed physicians much as they regarded teachers. Their basic duty was to function as learned theorists, and then most often in the surroundings of the aristocratic household.[98] Their learning and knowledge of many areas made them of value, but the Hellenistic physician's practice tended to follow his abstruse training in philosophical and medical opinions.[99] The Roman continued to reserve judgement for himself, even when he received advice from a doctor.

Medical theory and practice as they stemmed from the Hellenistic 'schools' were available to only a knowledgeable élite in the Roman Empire. In consequence, physicians had great difficulty communicating the base of their practice to their patients, and a few went so far as to make clear it was their intent not to do so. The public found itself alienated from medicine in its formal terms, and both Greek and Latin non-medical literature from the Empire reflect this estrangement. The aristocrats did, however, borrow the Hellenistic methods of contraception and showed again the Roman willingness to adapt Hellenistic ideas which led to practical results. Perhaps most importantly, the non-medical sources in their views of medicine show firmly the weakness of the overlay of Hellenism in the west, and the separation from the masses of the Hellenistic intellectual medicine in the east.

CHAPTER VIII

THE DOCTOR AND HIS PLACE IN ROMAN SOCIETY

DESPITE THE PUBLIC HUE about the poor performance of physicians in the Roman Empire, the best doctors commanded great prestige as they made their rounds and treated their patients. If the modern reader contemplates the negative statements of Pliny, Martial, Lucian, Plutarch, and the *Greek Anthology* in isolation, and assumes public opinion mirrors the actual social position of the physician, he is sadly misled. The knotty puzzle of the seeming rejection of the physician by the ordinary man, yet his acceptance by the leading elements in Roman society, can be solved only if the modern observer deals with Roman physicians on social and intellectual planes, rather than scientific ones. Roman public reaction points to a series of social distinctions, ranging from the absolute mistrust by the common man to the aristocratic adaptation of Hellenistic contraceptive methods.

Two conclusions appear to emerge from the evidence. If one accepts the positive statements from the medical writers themselves (Galen, Rufus, Aretaeus, and the rest), and the rare praise in the non-medical literature, he gains a view of a universally respected medicine in the Empire. If, on the other hand, one believes the caustic notices of ghosts cursing doctors, or the clever writer who pokes brutal fun at the doctor's vacuous prolixity, he seems to see a degenerate Greek or Hellenistic medicine as it existed in the Roman Empire. Both conclusions are common in the consideration of medicine among the Romans, but both ignore the Roman opinion of what medical practice entailed. Cato pointed the way to the ideal of the all-knowledgeable *pater familias,* and Celsus rounded it off in his masterly synthesis, still making the Roman the final judge of Hellenistic theories. Yet side by side with the Roman *medicus-pater familias* were countless Greek physicians who figure heavily in our sources. The practice of Soranus, Rufus, Aretaeus, and Galen is clear in its emphasis and direction, but the Greek assertions of medical knowledge do not seem to square with the usual physician-baiting common in imperial literature. A further deepening of the quandary results when the *medicus* of the legion proves to be one who learns his skill in the army, or when Roman aristocrats increasingly turn to self-care when access to Greek physicians is easy. With some care, we can sift the evidence and grasp the real role of the physician in Roman society. What we see in Galen is something akin to a philosopher-physician, and as such a man worked among the Romans, his efforts reflect the Roman concept of the worth of medicine.

Caesar and Augustus encouraged Hellenistic medicine in Rome with the same inducement Rome gave to the settlement of Greek teachers.[1] These foreign scholars received civic rights and Vespasian gave them freedom from civic responsibility. They also acquired the right to form associations of their own.[2] At first Hellenistic physicians came to Rome through the purchase of prisoners of war, particularly during the period of Roman expansion in the Hellenistic east to 146 BC. Noble Romans who could afford to purchase these highly educated individuals found they made valuable additions to their households, and they functioned as personal doctors in the homes of the aristocrats.[3] Many of the slave-physicians later obtained their freedom and set up practice of their own in Rome and were joined by numbers of Greek doctors who came to Rome on their own after 200 BC. Initially the Romans received them warmly, sometimes providing them with shops from which to conduct their practice.[4] Soon, however, the Romans became wary of them with a widespread mistrust. The reaction to Hellenistic medicine became quite bitter as the brutal invectives of Cato and Pliny emphasize.[5] Celsus tones down the blunt attacks on Hellenistic physicians, but his attempt to put order into the chaos of medical theories also reflects Roman reaction against Greek theory.[6] The Roman public understood only that Hellenistic doctors theorized a great deal and sometimes killed their patients while promising cure.

Even with the rejection on the part of the general populace, the Greek physician practised in sizeable numbers within the aristocratic households in the late Republic and Empire. The foreign doctor soon acquired a social distinction of his own. The physicians in personal service in the imperial house came to be examples of the status commanded in the social world of the early Empire.[7] The Roman aristocrats distinguished between what Hellenistic medicine could provide, and what could be expected from a *medicus*, whom the Romans knew as an 'ordinary' doctor who practised among the public.[8]

Within the Roman home, Hellenistic doctors were usually of the class of slaves or freedmen, and their function and duties present a puzzle to the modern observer who forgets the contempt of Galen. Inscriptions give some insight into the problem. Fifty doctors appear together in one section of the *CIL*, but only two are free-born foreigners beyond doubt.[9] Twelve are called freedmen and thirteen have only one name, indicating they were either slave or free. Of the rest, probably half were the descendants of freedmen. From this, one can formulate that about a quarter of the doctors in Rome were freedmen or their descendants.[10] Yet the most famous doctors were *peregrini* from the Hellenistic east. Charicles, the physician of Tiberius, was a free immigrant,[11] as were Andromachus the Cretan of Nero's day,[12] P. Stertinius Xenophon of Cos and his brother under Claudius,[13] and Galen in the second century. Antonius Musa, freedman of Antony and Augustus' physician, was a noteworthy exception to the rule,[14] but he received the right to wear a gold ring after he saved Augustus with cold baths. L. Arruntius Sempronianus designates himself one of the 'Asclepians' of Domitian,[15] and the physicians of Ephesus were proud of the patronage they received from the imperial house.[16] Hundreds of inscriptions, found throughout the Empire, give proof of freedman doctors,[17] but some became famous for their monstrous wealth rather than their skilled practice.[18] State pay for the luckier physicians probably was instituted

in the early Empire,[19] and the legal codes of the later Empire
preserved the tradition.[20] The remnants of the customary use of
physicians in the cities of the Empire suggest the class structuring
noted for the early Empire, as does a tidbit from the *Historia
Augusta*,[21] giving the impression of pay according to social rank.

Occasionally doctors appear as important political figures, who
had worked their way into positions of power. Criton, Trajan's
physician during the Dacian Wars, was the highly honoured
official historian for that difficult campaign.[22] An interesting case
is L. Gellius Maximus, who was a friend of Caracalla. He was an
archiatros and the son of a physician from Ephesus, and he led an
abortive attempt to capture the principate as the legate of the
Fourth Legion (Scythica), stationed in Syria. He was executed in
219.[23] Gellius apparently was one of an important group of politicians active in promoting the arts in Ephesus and Antioch, taking
a cue from Pergamon and its famous Museum.[24] In addition to
pursuing political ambitions, these doctors were the heads of
families which boasted about their philosophic and scientific skill,
and their influence at Antioch was long-lived.[25]

In the fourth century, a doctor attempted to make his influence
felt in Rome. Dorus had formerly been physician for the *scutarii*
and had risen in the ranks until he was promoted to command
Rome's night watch, which guarded the public buildings and
monuments. He was favoured by Magnentius and became involved
in one of the intrigues plaguing the city. He accused Adelphius,
Prefect of Rome, of having ambition for greater power, and the
matter came before one of the Emperor Constantius' investigating
committees. The intrigue had widened to include the accusations
brought against Arbetio, a former barbarian who had risen from
the ranks to be cavalry commander. Arbetio was consul in 355,
but a certain Verissimus, a rival for Arbetio's position, accused
Arbetio of aspiring to the purple. Verissimus and Dorus, the
doctor now turned plotter, hoped to gain from a common suit
against Arbetio and Adelphius. Dorus accused Arbetio as well,
and the two officials seemed doomed. Constantius apparently
directed his chamberlains to acquit Adelphius and Arbetio, and
the two accusers lost what position they had. Verissimus 'instantly

was silent' and Dorus 'evaporated', suggesting imperial wrath took their lives.[26]

The physician was politician as well as philosopher and the boldest were not afraid to enter the uncertain world of the army and imperial politics in the third and fourth centuries. Fame rested on attributes other than medical practice. The Hellenistic physicians ran the gamut of social classes, from slaves to companions to the Roman emperor, and we can speculate that many of these men were trained, as was Galen, who boasts of his philosophic background as often as he tells us of his medical skill.

The Romans viewed medicine as the province of slaves and freedmen. As medicine emerged from the Hellenistic world into the Roman Empire, its character did not attract a people who rather feebly displayed talents for the building of philosophical systems. Romans tended to snub the profession as practised by the Greeks. The mere dependence on the patient by the doctor for his diagnosis, and the personal contact a doctor had to have with his patients, pushed the Romans away from the practice of medicine.[27] Politician-physicians, philosopher-physicians, and the household *medicus* existed in the same era, and nobody felt they overlapped in their functions. Ammianus, speaking of the moral gloom of the fourth century in the Empire, notes that 'all the healing art is powerless' to help correct the problems,[28] and his observation tells us the regard that medicine received among aristocrats: it was an amalgam of philosophical tenets and scientific views, but it had no formal boundaries as we classify it today.

The rare praise physicians receive in the non-medical sources help us to understand the social puzzle of Roman medicine. Cicero grieves about the death of his free doctor Asclapon and his slave Alexion, not so much that he has lost good physicians, but that he was poorer for the loss of their humanity and charm.[29] Seneca provides the major example of the quality of man expected in a physician, as he speaks of the friendship he has with his doctor. 'Since they become friends from being a doctor and a teacher, and we owe them something, not particularly because of their skill, which they sell, but on account of their kindness and friendly attitude towards us.' Seneca learns from his doctor, not only the

H

skills of his profession, but something also of good character
which the best physicians exemplify.[30] The doctor who merely
'does his job', arrives at the summons of the patient, feels the
pulse, and gives advice on what to do or what to avoid, and
Seneca writes, 'I owe him nothing more.'[31] From this Seneca
distinguishes the man who renders advice from one who renders a
benefit,[32] and there are two kinds of physicians in Seneca's experience: those who know the methods and techniques of medicine,
and those who possess humanity, a thorough knowledge of
philosophy, and wide learning. Such as the latter Seneca wanted
to befriend, but the rest he ignored, as he did ferrymen. Seneca's
ideal doctor was a teacher too. The Roman was suspicious of the
physician who worked for pay, and felt the quest for wealth
warped judgement and hindered proper treatment.[33]

The philosopher-physician hailed from a long tradition of
medical theory, and considered the knowledge of Greek essential
in order to comprehend medicine at all. On occasion, Galen waxes
satirical about the ignorance of his fellows, and shows the dichotomy
between the philosopher-physician and the Roman citizen.

You think I ought to learn a number of languages, but I feel
it is proper to learn but one, that one which is my own. All
peoples can use it, and it is sweet-sounding and expressive for
all mankind. If, however, you want to master a language of
the barbarians, you would be wise to understand that some of
the barbarian tongues sound like noises that pigs, frogs, and
crows make, since they lack form and elegance, and are not
suited for the tongue, lips, and mouth. Almost always some
of these people speak deep in their throats as if they were
snoring, and they use their lips to hiss, or to make their voices
squeak, or to speak in a dreary tone; or they talk with gaping
mouth while they roll their tongues around, or they barely
open their mouths at all, and they appear to have tongues
without movement and immobile as if they were attached to
the mouth. . . . If you do not wish to learn Greek, then you
are a barbarian.[34]

Vogt sums the problem well as he writes, '. . . the scientific art of healing . . . was represented so arrogantly and opaquely by these Greeks, the politically conquered but the intellectually superior.'[35]

The learned physicians, such as Galen, who became common as doctors in the great households of the Empire, show training that Celsus does not exhibit except by indirect method.[36] There is little disputing that Galen represented the best of the medico-philosophical tradition from the Hellenistic world, but his early training demonstrates far more than medicine and its techniques. The physician was, in the first analysis, a learned man, well-schooled in philosophy and what we term the fine arts. Galen thinks of himself as a good judge of sculpture,[37] and proudly calls his father 'second to none of the philosophers'.[38] Young Galen studied various 'fields of knowledge'. His father felt Greek literature was the foundation, but valued the study of mathematics, architecture, astronomy, and agriculture.[39] Seed testing was among the pursuits in Galen's home-training with his father.[40] When Galen was fifteen, he became a student of an Epicurean, but his father urged him to take up medicine for practical reasons when he was eighteen.[41] None the less, Galen asserts that philosophy and medicine were equal in his career, and both commanded his enthusiasm.[42] When Galen began his medical studies, the revival of Hippocrates was in vogue, and he sat with various teachers in Pergamon, Smyrna, Corinth, and Alexandria.[43] He returned for a time to his home city, Pergamon, and became physician to the gladiators there.[44] Later (c. 162) Galen went to Rome to establish a reputation as a philosopher-physician.[45]

Galen's work showed the heavy influence of philosophy. The correlation of structure and function dominated his anatomical investigations, and to Galen this was the 'real base of the perfect theology which transcended all other aspects of medicine'.[46] This 'bright light'[47] guided his work in medicine. Analogies were important for Galen to draw conclusions. Children's education received principles from gardening,[48] and digestion was explained by the observation of the magnetic attraction of iron.[49] The world of botany gave Galen his description of the eye and the optic nerve: it was a poppy seed capsule.[50] Galen utilized comparative anatomy—the dissection of a crane and an ostrich—to prove the marvellous uniformity of the recurrent laryngeal nerve,[51] and his teleological tendencies became marked as he considered the expansive and contractive properties of the uterus.[52]

Galen performed public demonstrations of his skill in anatomy and surgery to establish himself in Rome. Later he was asked to repeat some of this before an audience of a few of the great names in Rome, including political leaders and others of the collected intellectuals deemed competent to watch and make comments. The list of those attending Galen's demonstrations reveals much about attitudes towards medicine and its practitioners. Present was Paulus, soon to become Prefect of Rome. The consular, Flavius, as well as a consul, Servius, were in attendance, representing the Roman government. Sergius was a high public official, and Barabarus was the uncle of Lucius Verus, who was then on an expedition in Mesopotamia. Adrian was a rhetorician, Demetrius an orator,[53] and the Peripatetic philosopher, Alexander of Damascus, would soon take up duties as a teacher in Athens.[54]

Among his public performances, Galen was proud of his demonstration of the structure and function of the organs of respiration and their relation to vocal sounds. He operated on a large pig in a well-lit room, and he paralysed the intercostal muscles with ligatures, thus stilling the squalling animal. Galen then released the ties and caused great wonder among the spectators as the pig took up its loud squealing again.[55] Galen was seeking an answer to the function of respiration and the possible link to voice production. He based his conclusions upon the medico-philosophical concepts bequeathed to him.[56] Probably many of the dissections were directed by Galen, and assistants (slaves?) did the actual cutting. At one point Galen became disgusted at their efforts and ended up doing much of the work himself.[57]

Galen spent his career in Rome as one of the learned philosopher-physicians and he attended to the needs of Marcus Aurelius and his son Commodus.[58] His prolific writing demonstrates his predilection for philosophy as well as the amalgam of the objective and the irrational characteristic of his age.[59] Galen's *Introduction to Logic* exhibits peculiarities, marking it as Stoic, Peripatetic, and being of no traditional philosophical school, and appears to be a milestone in the history of ancient philosophy for its originality and eclecticism.[60] His impact upon the Arabs was profound in both philosophy and medicine.[61] Sambursky gives Galen full credit for the 'qualitative theory of matter' which was the rule in science for 1,500 years.[62] Galen introduced a great measure of flexibility into the concepts of the qualities of matter and gave rise to a long-standing system of terminology for biology and medicine.[63] Galen's goal was to retain the sensory links with these concepts and to attempt to build physical standards for them so that they could be measured.[64]

Problems came as Galen sought to standardize the four qualities and the resulting mixture of terms shows the problem of concise scientific terminology in antiquity.[65] Ambiguity reigned as Galen attempted to be precise about warmth, coolness, and the like. But proportion was another of those factors which allowed the Greek genius full play in aesthetic achievement, and symmetry and balance were focal concepts in the Greek and Hellenistic scientific mind. Galen, in one of his analogies, clarifies this for us. Painters and those who work in stone attempt to portray the most beautiful of each type, such as the most beautifully created man, horse, bull, or lion, and the artist seeks the mean of every type.[66] Likewise, the physician had to look for the mean, or proportional qualities, in his diagnosis.[67] In raising the question of quantitative definition of a pastiche of qualities, Galen posed problems that the Greco-Roman ideal could not solve, and he was forced to borrow from the standard philosophic bank for his terms and definitions.

Galen accepted the old doctrine of four elements (fire, air, earth, water) as corresponding to the four humours of the human body, that is blood, black bile, yellow bile, and phlegm. He received his concept of the humours from Aristotle and Hippocrates,[68] and proportion was important to Galen as he sought explanation for health and diseases.[69] The *crasis*, or mixture, of the elements and humours in correct ratios to one another gives health, and an improper blending gives sickness to the body.[70] Galen also believed the Platonic doctrine of the three souls who ruled yet

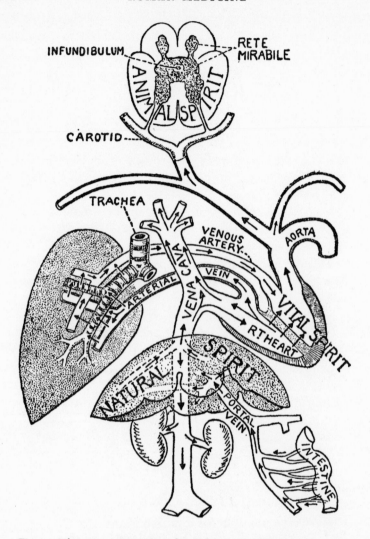

Fig. 13 Schematic representation of Galen's concept of physiology, or what we label physiology (vide note 68, p. 216)

served the body. The three lived in the heart, brain, and liver, and Galen classed them as the choleric, rational, and sensual souls. The choleric soul ruled passion and provided the vital force, the rational soul gave reason and thought with sensation and motion, and the sensual soul provided nutrition—hence the 'vegetative soul'. All three were but part of the one soul which lives in the body and Galen was not quite sure what its final substance could be termed.[71] The agents of the soul were the various *pneumata*, and there were two basic kinds. Air entering the lungs was changed subtly so that it could enter a vein and mingle with blood. In the vein the mixture was altered to become proto-*pneuma*, which in turn became *pneuma* after going from the lungs via veins to the left ventricle of the heart and combining with more blood which seeped into the chamber from the right ventricle through assumed pores in the interventricular septum. Now vital *pneuma* was driven into the arteries and distributed throughout the body. The blood on its way to the brain underwent another transformation. Galen thought that before the carotid arteries carried the vital *pneuma* to the brain, it passed through a complicated network of vessels (the *rete mirabile*)[72] that aided the work of the brain which changed the vital *pneuma* into psychic *pneuma*. The new transformation came with the aid of air from the ventricles via the olfactory bulbs. Psychic *pneuma*, which was altered air and fed by arterial blood, is called by Galen 'exhalation of useful blood'.[73] The psychic *pneuma* was then sent out through the invisible lumen of the nerves to provide sensation and motion. The optic nerves needed so much psychic *pneuma* that their lumen was the only visible one for the nerves, showing as hollow tubes.[74] Galen was not so sure about a third *pneuma*, a 'natural *pneuma*', which he thought might reside in the liver and the veins.[75]

Following his pattern of proportion in physiological theories, Galen supposed each division of the soul had a particular power along with its *pneuma*.[76] Further, Galen thought each of the body's organs had the power to attract the appropriate kind of nourishment to itself. Once the attraction had been exercised, then the balancing force, or the 'retentive faculty', began its operation. Galen extended this system of balancing forces to all of the body functions, mentioning various faculties taking command of the functions under consideration.[77]

Magic had great appeal in an age of dissolving religions, and much that came from Pythagoreanism was labelled simply 'magical numbers' in the Roman Empire. Galen denies the use of Pythagorean mystical numbers, noting the seven mouths of the Nile or the seven stars of the Pleiades had nothing to do with the crisis of the seventh day of inflammation in the chest or lungs.[78] After all, the critical point occurs often on the fourth, fifth, ninth, and tenth days.[79] But Galen accepted magical charms and amulets as having some power, and tells us green jasper helps take care of abdominal pains, but he feels the prescription of King Nechepsos —which he quotes—is wrong. One can use the charm without the engraving of a snake and a star-wreath.[80] Galen deemed astrology as one of the great discoveries of the Egyptian astronomers, and believed the moon's position in the good and evil planets had great power over the condition of his patients.[81] Diseases were particularly troublesome if the good stars were in Aries, and the bad stars in Taurus, and the moon in Taurus, Leo, Scorpio, or Aquarius, at the birth of a patient. But diseases were mild for the patient who was born when the moon was crossing Aries, Cancer, Libra, or Capricorn.[82] Galen further asserts that someone who 'refused to observe these matters or refused to believe in the observation of others, was an undoubted sophist who noisily shouts down other opinions, and who postulates reasons for the apparent, and who does not attempt to go from known phenomena to hidden things.'[83] His conclusions on the use of astrology come in terms understood by the student of philosophy.

Galen lived and worked within the matrix of the higher intellectual circles of Rome, which included rhetoricians, grammarians, philosophers, legal experts, orators, architects, astrologers, and even athletes.[84] His duties were to attend to the needs of the royal house, prescribe remedies for various illnesses, and to discuss matters of intellectual import at the behest of the royal court and its inhabitants. Drug prescriptions were numerous and complicated,[85] and philosopher-physicians did not understand why drugs worked (if they did) any more than the *medici* or the *iatroliptai*.[86]

The Hellenistic physician arrived in Rome as a portion of the complexity of Greek philosophy, and the Roman recognized this kind of 'doctor' in a special way.[87] Galen was ranked on a par with others of the intellectual élite and teachers of many fields. Galen and his medical colleagues were highly valued, but among the aristocrats alone. Some Greek physicians were available to the masses but we hear about them caustically through Galen and many examples in Plutarch, Lucian, and the *Greek Anthology*. The *medicus* appears in our sources only indirectly, with the exception of the legions, and he is the Latin counterpart of the ignorant, over-talkative Greek physician recruiting his patients on the street. The drug dealer probably doubled as a *medicus* on occasion,[88] and his social rank is that of a shoemaker.[89] Yet the Roman *medicus* rises to the plane of a Celsus, and *medici* offer opinions to those who inquire of medical matters from them.[90] Sometimes the *medicus* merely watches the patient for a time and offers the results of his observations.[91] A good Roman education included knowledge of medicine as well as oratory and the rest.[92]

Our records, in particular Galen, speak eloquently of the philosopher-physician in residence in the aristocratic homes of the Empire. But their services were limited, and the common man had little access to the philosopher-physicians: they were too expensive. Doctors' fees became legends in their own time. Manilius Cornutus, ex-praetor and legate of Aquitania, agreed to the sum of 200,000 sesterces to be paid to a physician for treatment of a disease that left nasty scars.[93] Charmis of Massilia gained 200,000 sesterces by 'selling' one of his rich patients to a certain Alcon, the wound specialist.[94] Galen received 400 gold pieces from the consular, Boethus, for curing his wife.[95] Consultation by letter allowed the doctor to take his fee even when he could not visit his patients.[96] Rich patients often gave difficulty to the physician, but Galen assures us that they need to be endured.[97]

Galen ridicules the physician who goes among the people, assuming they are too stupid to understand his brand of medicine.

... if ... you should tell me of such things as are uttered by the man in the street, you would say nothing of men of quality ... you would be setting forth the information of the lower and less intelligent class of the inhabitants.[98]

CHAPTER IX

ROMAN MEDICAL EDUCATION

CLASSICAL EDUCATION took the individual as its ideal, and did not equip technicians for specialized functions, as we view 'education' in the twentieth century. Our age is characterized by an overwhelming fragmentation of knowledge which Greek and Roman thought deliberately denied.[1] The Romans were much aware of the possibilities of technical development, but chose to mould their ideal in a different path. As Marrou has noted in his admirable study, we cannot simply 'explain away' the lack of technical development in antiquity by noting the existence of slavery, but must attempt to 'understand it' by examining the ideals of classical education.[2]

Medicine developed into an autonomous branch of learning, almost uniquely among the various sciences in antiquity, because it had a 'more immediate social relevance.'[3] Even within its specialized activity, the best Roman physicians were haunted by a kind of inferiority complex. Galen says what Hippocrates had said before him, that the ideal physician must be a philosopher too.[4] The doctor had no wish to be isolated from his society, and medicine was part of the general culture. Medicine's enormous prestige has not returned in the modern United States owing to the severe specialization in the medicine of the twentieth century operating on a different plane than its inspirational counterpart in Greece and Rome. Roman medicine preserved the concept of medical practice which was a close relative of the ethical science of Socrates.[5] Jaeger gives it credit for being a leading cultural force in the system of classical ideals, and those ideals gave the modern world its view of the 'general education' of man. Medical science, as such, was created by the inspiration derived from the rediscovery of Greco-Roman ideals in medicine tempered with the Age of Reason.

The results of Galen's probings into anatomy and physiology mislead the modern reader who puts Galen into a 'scientific' context Galen would not have understood. More important for the understanding of the Greco-Roman medical ideal are the motivations which drove Galen into the path of dissection and experimentation. Galen laid his groundwork by rejecting the Epicurean-Asclepiadean tradition of an irrational Nature, and assumed a systematic, functional, teleological formation of organs.[6] None the less, he often reveals an unease about medical speculation, and tries to reconcile the realism of Aristotle with the idealism of Plato.[7] This was the backdrop of medical teaching in the Roman Empire: the conflict of theory and practice seen in Plato and Aristotle.[8] His anxiety led Galen into observation and experiment, offering results for settling doubts, but he voiced conclusions in terms of accepted philosophic constructs. Galen's creative imagination was not typical, and his ventures to find physiological significance of various parts of the body[9] often blind us to the fact that most physicians ignored experimentation. Galen had a happy facility of finding expression in analogy, and when he states 'sound is carried like a wave',[10] or something in the atmosphere acts in burning as it does in breathing,[11] we should not assume he had 'stumbled' into revolutionary discoveries: these are random thoughts of a complex and fertile mind moulded in the universal classical ideal. Galen 'knew his classics, could speak like a rhetor, and argue like a philosopher.'[12]

Plato in his *Laws* allows us to glimpse something of the ideal education of the physician, but we must note the difference between slave and free, practical and theoretical. 'One kind of doctor treats us in one fashion, another will use another . . . they have two different ways.' Plato then speaks of 'doctors and doctors' helpers' and labels them both 'doctors'. Both sorts obtain their learning in their skill under direction of an experienced physician, and the novices can either be free-born or slave. The acquired skill comes from 'observation and practice, not by the study of nature', but the free-born doctor has learned his art by the observation of nature and in this *he* can instruct his students. Plato, in his ideal, distinguishes two classes of doctors: doctors and doctors' slaves. The slave can learn at the behest of his medical master the techniques for treatment of other slaves and he can 'go around town treating other servants.' Meanwhile, the free-born doctor treats other freemen by a combination of reason, specula- tion, and medical experience, in a fashion that Plato describes as 'rational and humane.' The slave, although he may be 'trained', merely 'prescribes.'[13] Plato concludes this section of his *Laws* by noting that both methods in combination are better than the rational alone, or the prescribing alone.

Aristotle, on the other hand, notes that 'the science of nature' forms the background of the education of physicians.[14] He speaks of *three* kinds of doctors in his time, all of whom have skill and ability to practise. There is the craftsman, that is the ordinary practitioner, the 'specialist who directs the course of treatment', and the person 'who has studied the art.'[15] Then Aristotle adds, rather significantly, 'there are men of this last type to be found in connection with nearly all the arts; and we credit them with the power of judging as much as we do the experts—i.e. the practi- tioners and the experts.'[16]

Greek culture taught the importance of the body as well as the soul. The cosmopolitanism of the Hellenistic period is signalled by the development of gymnastics and the role of medicine. In descriptions of physical training in Plato and later, the doctor takes his place beside the trainer. Most men 'are ignorant of what is good or bad for the body . . . unless he is a trainer or a doctor.'[17] There were men 'who appear to be in good health that it is not easy for someone who is not a doctor or a trainer to know through observation that they are in poor health.'[18] Matters dealing with impurities of the body are 'successfully determined by medicine and gymnastics.'[19] For men and their problems, two skills (*duo technai*) existed which could help in two evil conditions (*duo pathemata*) of the body: 'for deformity there is gymnastics, and for disease there is medicine.'[20] In his ideal state Plato combined gymnastics and medicine into one study,[21] and in later develop- ment of Hellenistic and Roman medicine, the two were never far apart.[22] Within the intellectual areas, as a parallel, the philosopher appeared beside the musician and the poet.[23]

Celsus reconciles the conflict he sees in medical ideals and training, but he acknowledges that philosophers were the first experts in medicine.[24] He, like Aristotle, divided medicine up into what it could do, but in a different pattern. The Art was composed of three parts: diet, cures through medicaments, and surgery.[25] But Celsus doubts whether the long-lived philosophical ideal was the most important part of medicine. 'Even philosophers could be the greatest medical practitioners if syllogism could provide skill; in these matters they have words in great multitude, but no knowledge of healing,'[26] and adds, 'he who does not talk very much but who learns to observe things carefully will make a better doctor than the man who talks too much without medical experience.'[27] Later he admits medicine 'is a skill based on conjecture',[28] but the doctor's reasoning will aid his patient in the case of an unknown disease by the observation of apparent causes as well as a clear knowledge of the personal life of the patient.[29] Celsus nevertheless reaffirms the social importance of medicine to the educated Roman as he points out 'the doctor is more useful to you if he is a friend than if he is a stranger.'[30]

Medical education in Rome thus came to reflect the classical ideal inherited from the Hellenistic world, coupled with the strong assertion that the educated Roman could learn medicine. The sentiment is clearly expressed in Oribasius, as he says

It is desired, or really a necessity, that everyone should study medicine from youth alongside other fields and hear its principles, so that they can become good advisers in everything that is related to public safety.[31]

Within Greco-Roman medicine, practised by such as Celsus and Galen, medical education usually took the form of the practical training of a son as a doctor by his doctor father. This training operated in an unorganized fashion apart from any so-called school, sect, guild, library, or cult.[32] Of course the quality of instruction would vary but doctors came to label themselves Dogmatics, Methodists, and so forth simply because their fathers had

done so, without any real knowledge of the philosophic or metho-
dological issues involved.[33] The unease of the function of medicine
within Roman imperial society underlay the opposition of the so-
called Dogmatics and Empiricists. This conflict represented in
several ways the clash between theory and practice in medical
practice and education. Roman medicine at its best did not
encourage the specialization expected in modern scientific
medicine.

Surgery, because of its complete dependence upon knowledge
gained from actual experience, showed this conflict sharply as it
attempted to make its educational principles clear.

> For is it not absurd that a student who doesn't know what
> cataract, dropsy, etc., are, and does not understand the
> simplest matters in surgery, e.g. the different types of dress-
> ings and the uses of sponges, should concern himself with
> moot problems and inquire: What is surgery? How was it
> discovered? Is it better than dietetics? These questions are not
> pressing. They are extraneous problems for the scholar and
> should be reserved for later. But the students ought to be
> trained in the principles proper to surgery.[34]

Galen devotes much of his writing to outline some of these
principles—both of surgery and 'moot questions'—and uses the
opportunity to point up the differences of opinion among practitioners.[35] Some appear to be set pieces for public discussion, as
'How Was Medicine Discovered?', and the like. Galen as well as
Lucian tell of the uselessness of these dialectical disputes and
comment on their participants' lack of real medical knowledge.[36]

Medical education in the Roman world was haphazard, as our
sources indicate. Occasionally instruction would be given in
practical medicine by a teacher who took students with him as he
visited patients, or would offer medical lessons at his own shop,
the well-known *taberna medica*.[37] Sometimes towns built structures, something like the earlier Greek *iatreia*, to attract doctors to
settle,[38] and supplied them with surgical tools and various medical
appliances. Galen, in a long section,[39] has left us a rather complete
(and undoubtedly one of the most prolix and verbose) description

of such buildings: they were large with high doors, and had many windows which let in air and light. The sickrooms provided by the aristocratic Romans for their great households probably gave learning opportunities for the practical instruction, particularly if the slaves were ordered to learn medical skills by their master.[40] We hear of doctors' helpers and apprentices who accompanied their instructor when he went to see his patients,[41] but we also read of charlatans, such as Thessalus, who attracted many students by promising a complete medical education in six months. Thessalus supposedly made doctors of cooks, dyers, cobblers, fullers, and spinners in this short time.[42] Pliny may have someone like Thessalus in mind as he mutters his complaint at the lack of regulation of doctors in Rome.[43] On top of all this Galen tells us that most doctors in his day could not read.[44]

Lucian, in his *Disowned Son*, gives us various clues as to how one 'went into medicine' in the Roman Empire. His hero first states that he had 'devoted himself to the highest of callings', and he had gone abroad to study under the most famous doctors in foreign lands, and had 'through hard work and persistent enthusiasm mastered the skill of medicine'. Formerly he was an ordinary man, but now he was a doctor, and he was proud of his achievement in mastery of the complexities of medicine. At the same time Lucian's character asserts that the doctor, by the very nature of his profession, has freedom of movement and freedom to choose whom he treats. He notes that his medical education was given to him by distinguished doctors who taught sometimes for a fee, sometimes not.

Lucian's doctor learned something of pharmaceuticals, the humours, the differences in diseases between men and women,[45] but no indication is given of anatomy or the Galenic ideal of physiological experiment. Lucian respects the physician, particularly in his shrewd judgement when to and when not to treat diseases,[46] as well as the preponderant social prestige which he held among his fellows. Galen fills this picture out for us as he explains that doctors cannot learn anatomy from books[47]— implying they were available—nor can he learn from superficial observation of the body and its parts. Only in rare instances can the doctor actually observe such things as the movements of the heart in the human being, as he had done in a case of a thorax wound of a young boy.[48] To learn anatomy, the physician resorted to dissection of lower animals, such as the 'ape.'[49] Anatomy, according to Galen, was an absolute necessity for the physician,[50] but opportunities for human dissection were rarely available.[51] For the good physician, the reliance upon animal parallels, gained through personal dissection, was essential.[52] But Galen knew the doctor usually had little knowledge of anatomy, and wrote his *Anatomical Procedures* as an instruction-book in hopes to meet the deficiency.[53] Aulus Gellius probably consulted one of these handbooks as he 'boned up' on arteries and veins.[54]

Given the hit-and-miss approach of Roman medical education, and the irregular methods of recruitment into the profession, the best doctors attained remarkable insight. Pulse-lore became well developed in the diagnosis of various diseases.[55] Heart sounds may have been used for diagnostic purposes,[56] and leprosy, diarrhoea, jaundice, and tuberculosis were recognized as separate diseases.[57] Aretaeus describes what appears to be diphtheritic ulcer of the throat and mouth and terms it the 'Syrian or Egyptian Ulcer.'[58] Something of the pathology of the nervous system was known. Galen understood the connection between paralysis of the fingers and injury to the spinal column,[59] and Aretaeus apparently knew of the crossover of nervous fibres soon after their origin, explaining that when one side of the brain is damaged, the opposite side of the body is paralysed.[60] This list could be lengthened greatly, but shows that the best of Roman doctors performed well, even with the limitations imposed upon them in the classical ideal.

The doctor was charged with educating himself in another important aspect of his practice: drugs and 'pharmacology.' The most famous attempt to make some kind of order out of great confusion is the handbook of Dioscorides, who collected his data while he was a soldier under Lucilius Bassus.[61] Dioscorides is highly valued by Galen,[62] and notes that the physician must know botany and 'pharmacology.' He has to know all the plants, or at least 'those most used in medicines', and the doctor should study the various stages of growth in these plants, so that he can 'observe

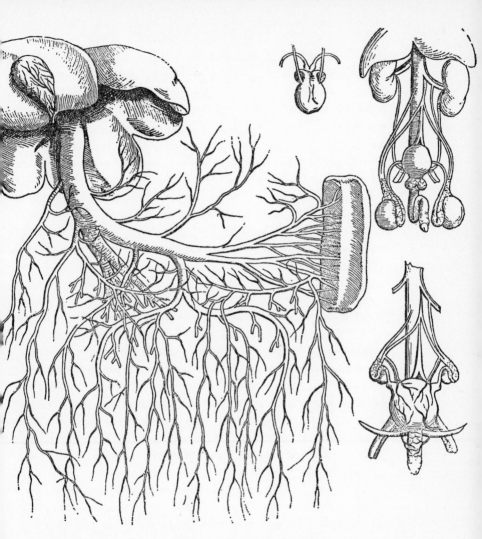

14 *Vesalius' concept of Galenic portal circulation. He had dissected cadavers and seen the [por]tal system for himself yet Galen's influence remained predominant. The liver pictured is [sch]ematized from Galenic animal anatomy, but Vesalius indicates his awareness of the bi-lobed [hu]man liver (inset, upper right) as contrasted to the five-lobed diagram, left. The small [dra]wing (top, centre) is probably the bladder, prostate, deferent ducts, ampullae, and ureters [(wr]ongly) of a dog. Note the 'cornua' on the uterus (lower right) and the analogy with the [pro]state gland in the male organs (upper right). The Galenic tradition af analogy (here [par]allels between male and female sex organs) is most important to Vesalius (vide Singer, [P]rocedures, preface, and J. B. de C. M. Saunders,* Vesalius: The Illustrations, *p. 237).*

I

that plants and fruits brought from Crete can also be found in the neighbourhood of Rome.'[63] Again Galen states it is impossible to learn botany from books, and the doctor has to learn the plants by patiently hunting them, preferably under the direction of an experienced teacher.[64] Botany books were available for instruction, as Pliny writes, with gross confusion in the illustrations,[65] but the physician and medical students had to observe plants often 'in order to gain a thorough knowledge of them.'[66]

Drug fraud gave physicians grave problems. The common practice was to rely upon drug dealers for supply. Pliny chuckles at how easily doctors were fooled by worthless concoctions as doctors in his day no longer made their own but were governed by names in handbooks of prescriptions.[67] Galen shows great concern over being cheated by drug dealers, and attempted to avoid them altogether by making long journeys to obtain genuine material, and had drugs sent to him from abroad by reliable contacts.[68] Galen says he studied under a 'learned corrector of fraudulent drugs' in his youth, who taught him the secrets of his trade for a large fee,[69] but notes that drug frauds are done with such skill that even experts could be fooled.[70] Worthless mixtures were brought into Rome by vendors from the surrounding countryside, and they, not the usual drug dealers, were the worst offenders.[71] The prescriptions were often long and complicated. Theriaca, for example, consisted of more than 70 animal and vegetable products.[72]

Although the Roman physician was forced to educate himself in many respects, there is reasonably good evidence showing that a few of the handbooks in medicine became standard by the later Empire. Galen, Hippocrates, and commentaries were used at Alexandria, long after its great days of dissection.[73] It is probable that most physicians did not have personal access to books or illustrative drawings, but the respected centres of medical study kept collections for reference. Alexandria's repute survived even in the day of Ammianus Marcellinus,[74] and the library figured in Ammianus' statement, 'medical studies at Alexandria go on expanding, although the doctor's work is poor. . . .' A good guess would suggest that medical students went to Alexandria to consult the collection under the direction of professors *before* they launched into private practice.

Similar to the standardized works available for consultation were those few which were written explicitly as instruction manuals for use in medicine. Galen wrote his *Anatomical Procedures, On the Dissection of Muscles for Amateurs,* and the *On Bones for Amateurs,* among many others, to meet the demand for clear guidebooks.[75] Galen says he responded to the requests of his colleagues when he wrote *Muscles,* as 'there had just been received a prolix summary of 15,000 lines (with errors to match) done up by Lycus. . . . My book is but a third as long, but I clearly outline all the muscles. . . . Anyone can gain for himself experience by dissecting an ape with my book before him. . . .'[76] Something of the medical ideal, and the close ties between gymnastics and medicine, becomes clear in Galen's *On the Protection of Health.* This treatise shows the problems of handbooks as Galen writes, 'a few doctors and trainers who have written certain books on the protection of health proposed hypotheses applicable to everyone, without thinking of the differences in the types of our bodies. . . . In my first book I outlined clearly how there are many types of human bodies . . . and instructed according to the assumption of perfect health in youth and how the young man should be brought up. . . .'[77] Soranus wrote his *Gynecology* as a guidebook for midwives and divided his subject into two sections: one on the midwife, and the second on the things with which the midwife is faced.[78] Doubtlessly these kinds of textbooks formed the bulk of the collections at the great medical libraries at Pergamon, Smyrna, and Alexandria, and the prospective physician received instruction from them. Probably there was no regular preparation of doctors within the temples to Asclepius, as they were devoted to other means of healing.[79]

Physicians apparently attempted to regulate themselves by formation of medical clubs which had quarters of their own as well as secretaries to record proceedings of meetings.[80] The right to form such *collegia medicorum* was especially granted by imperial decree,[81] and may form the backbone of the tradition embedded in later regulations in the *Codex Theodosianus* regarding physicians and their social role and their teaching responsibilities.[82] Medical teachers were granted stipends, but our evidence is from the later Empire and by no means completely reliable.[83] By the time of Constantine, salaries for doctors form a section of the complicated regulations of the changing Roman world, and the doctor still retains the association with others of the intellectual community and is a part of the general ideal of 'teacher'.[84]

The gymnasium found in all major cities of the eastern half of the Empire outwardly symbolized Hellenistic education and the Greek way of life. The office of gymnasiarch carried with it some expense as well as honour.[85] The major cost was the oil for the members of the gymnasium, young and old.[86] Generally the burden of the office was heavy, particularly in the large cities. The major support for education did not come from direct payment to teachers but rather by the granting of remission of municipal burdens. The remission was partial in the case of elementary teachers and complete for doctors and lawyers. Again we see the welding of the gymnastic with the medical, and the chief function of the city was to provide facilities for their practice.[87] Antoninus Pius established a given number of physicians who would be available to the various cities according to their sizes: ten for the largest, seven for middle-sized cities, and five for the smaller centres.[88] These doctors received a salary from the state for giving medical instruction and treating the poor without fees.

Numerous inscriptions from Ephesus indicate that there was a Museum there, organized on the model of Alexandria. To it was attached an association of physicians,[89] and medical studies and techniques were encouraged through public contests. The older, more experienced physicians competed for prizes by writing essays on surgery, the public display of surgical skill with instruments, and solving problems given by the judges for solution on the spot.

Training and recruitment in Roman medicine operated from the informal base of the tradition of a family, apprenticeship, and the collecting of books at well-known centres of medical instruction. The rise of groups of physicians in 'sects' shows that medical education, as such, reflected some inner unease at the scientific nature of the physician's duties as opposed to the cultural ideal of the time. Important for the future of medicine is the separation of surgery and medicine, as defined by Celsus. Likewise the acceptance of written works of Greek and Roman medicine had long-range implications: the best work of the physicians could be studied by future generations, who would not experiment in the pattern of Rufus and Galen. In turn these 'medical classics' became the standards for Arabic and later medieval medicine and, upon re-examination, gave the spark of the fantastic anatomical and medical activity in the Renaissance. Perhaps the most important facet of Roman medical education, with its practical and theoretical sides, was the combination of rational approaches in medicine, carrying on the great breakthrough of the Ionian philosophers of old.

CHAPTER X

THE EFFECTIVENESS
OF ROMAN MEDICINE
IN ROMAN SOCIETY

ROME KNIT HER EMPIRE into a cosmopolitan whole and she created symbols of her effective rule which reached into the personal life of every citizen. Aqueducts, baths, public works of many kinds attested to the gigantic amalgam that allowed the Empire to function. Public welfare formed a major consideration of the Roman rule, and effective means were found to deal with public waste, public water supply, and to some degree with public welfare. A basic humanity pervaded legal Roman approaches to medical and social problems in the long period reaching from the Twelve Tables to Ulpian.[1] Rome inherited a long tradition of competent care for the needy from the Hellenistic world,[2] and she gradually adopted programmes of her own, coming under the heading of *alimenta* by the reign of Nerva.[3] The coinage of the second century reflected Rome's pride in her manner of caring for her poor, and formed an important piece of Rome's image which she wished her subjects to respect and admire.[4] Within the system as it stood in its first two centuries, the citizen recognized a stable and efficient pattern in his relations with the government. With the exception of the imperial political structure, the Roman perceived his right to freedom of opinion on many aspects of his personal life as they brushed against the public bustle. Doctors and patients had views in this fashion, and some of the recorded reflections of the time allow us to judge something of the rather intangible level of effectiveness of medicine in the Roman Empire.

Many patients reacted with disapproval to the professional physician in the Empire, but this is only one aspect in considering the effectiveness of medicine. Side by side with the non-medical sources, the medical literature of the day contains fascinating sketches of medicine's relation with the public at large as well as what physicians themselves felt to be normal accomplishment. Again we must exercise extreme care in the analysis of ancient 'concepts' of science. We need to note the prodigious influence of magic and the traditional forms of religious medical practice upon both doctors and their patients. Most doctors believed in dreams and the best of them valued amulets, yet their surgery and treatment was not irrational nor unscientific in historic context. The patients in the Empire did not feel their services to be more incompatible with temples of Asclepius than is the use of Medicare with fascination for best-selling paperbacks on American folk recipes or the traditional farmer's almanac.[5] Roman medicine had brilliantly synthesized the aspects of medicine in the classical tradition to include the rational elements of the Hippocratic 'school', the short-lived Alexandrian experiments, the Roman gentleman's learned and simple solution, as well as astrology, religious medicine, magic, and folk traditions older than organized culture. Roman medicine knew its limits and recognized things which by argument and reason were unknown but which doctors could not avoid or 'hold aloof from because they have a being which is not evident.'[6] Galen admitted the existence of matters which he could not 'understand', but which medicine in one of its varied forms could elucidate.[7]

Modern studies in anthropology and zoology provide some intriguing conclusions which bear on the problem of the Roman medical definition. Although such terms as 'social grooming' and 'grooming talk' may allow us to chuckle at the imprecision of the scientists and their vocabulary, the concept is important for the understanding of ancient medicine. Morris, in his recent *The Naked Ape*, attempts to give some coherence to the 'non-human' traits he sees in man. For Morris, medical practice grew out of social grooming behaviour among the primates,[8] with the first step being simple skin care accompanied by 'grooming talk'.[9] Morris views the modern medical world as a 'condition of complexity that [is] . . . the major expression of animal comfort behaviour.'[10] In probing beneath the surface of modern technical and rational medicine, with its unique achievements, there appear many irrational elements. General practitioners of the twentieth century are well aware of the problem that Morris raises in the distinction between serious and trivial cases of indisposition. To be sure, man becomes infected by parasites or breaks an arm on a purely accidental basis, but most sicknesses are not what they appear to be. Minor illnesses receive rational treatment as if they are 'simply versions of serious illnesses but there is strong evidence to suggest that they are in reality much more related to primitive grooming demands. The medical symptoms reflect a behavioural problem that has taken a physical form, rather than a true physical problem.'[11] Morris calls coughs, colds, backache, headache, skin rashes, sore throats, and the like 'grooming invitation illnesses' and that the 'exact nature of the chemicals prescribed is almost irrelevant and there is little difference at this level between the practices of modern medicine and those of ancient witch-doctoring.'[12]

One may differ with Morris's blanket inclusion, but the idea is worth reflection. Roman medicine was superb in its rational treatment of many ills, which the modern physician might describe as trivial. The Romans, none the less, understood well that level of medicine which was 'psychosomatic', and which was best performed in the social or intellectual context. Here the Roman physician possessed a self-assurance and mastery which Galen, Aretaeus, Soranus, and Celsus unconsciously displayed. The cogency of Roman medicine was its proficiency in dealing with most problems of medicine, and providing solutions which were accepted within the age. Aelius Aristides' search for medical help painfully indicated the Roman citizen's need for the intimate care which Asclepius, rather than the physicians, gave. The Roman did not call his approach to medicine 'psychological', yet he commanded a full understanding of cures for the sort of medical problems Morris terms trivial, and, at the same time, gave organization and meaning to medicine on many levels, from the scholar-physician to the magic amulets sold in Egypt. Galen's massive work capped

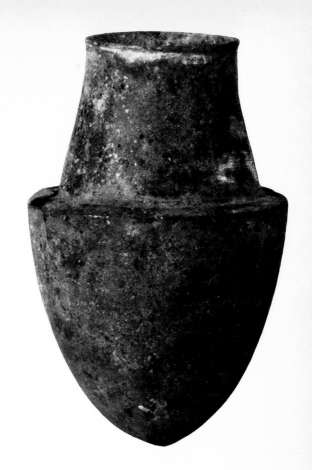

38 Bronze cupping
vessel from Corfu. This
example, 4.6 in. high, is a
typical one and serves to
show how greatly
enlarged, and therefore
symbolic, is the
specimen seen on the
stele of Jason, Plate 37.
(Celsus, II, 11,
Oribasius VII, 16).
British Museum.

39 Group of bronze instruments showing a syringe (nasal?), forceps, flat probe,
salve scoop, small mixing bowl and bone forceps. British Museum.

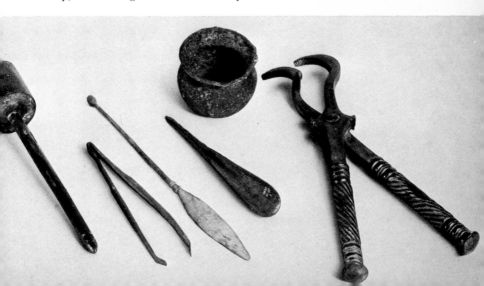

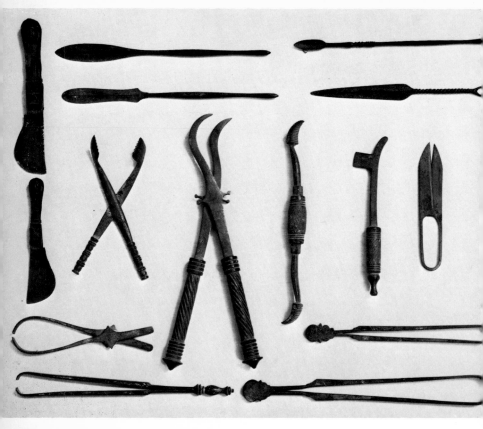

40 Various bronze instruments from Pompeii found in houses other than the 'House of the Surgeon.' Included here are scalpels (left), variants on the basic form of a flat probe (top), 'uvula' forceps (centre, left; Paul of Aegina VI, 21, 79), bone forceps (centre), bone lever or rasp probe, lancet (?), surgical scissors, polyp forceps (all centre, right) and, below, four examples of forceps including a hinged pair. Naples Museum.

41 Above left, an ornate, but bent, probe; below, a fine-toothed bone saw; right, a salve spreader or tongue depressor, and closed 'uvula' forceps. British Museum.

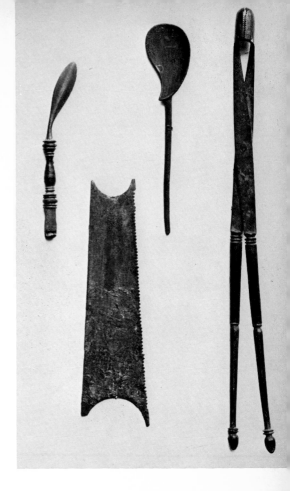

42 Three examples of bronze spatulae having shapes that suggest their function. Below, the broad, flat blade is suitable for spreading thick salves; centre and top, round-ended spatulae probably for use in spreading thinner salves over wide areas. British Museum.

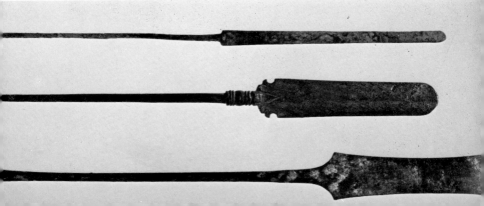

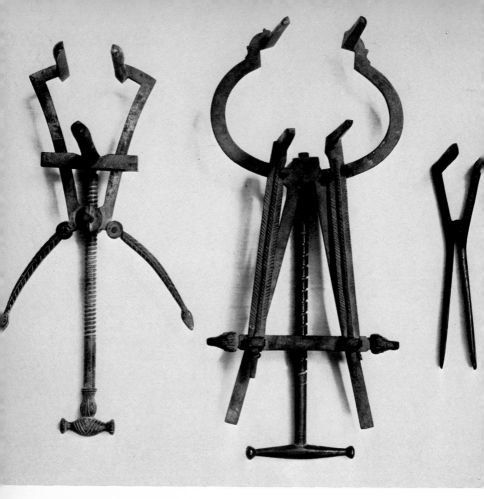

43 Different kinds of vaginal specula, ranging from a basic screw mechanism for opening to a more complicated arrangement allowing a finer adjustment, centre. Right, a plainer example, probably typical of that used by the ordinary doctor or midwife. These instruments show a sophistication of manufacture and the first two were probably not in common use in the Empire due to their expense.

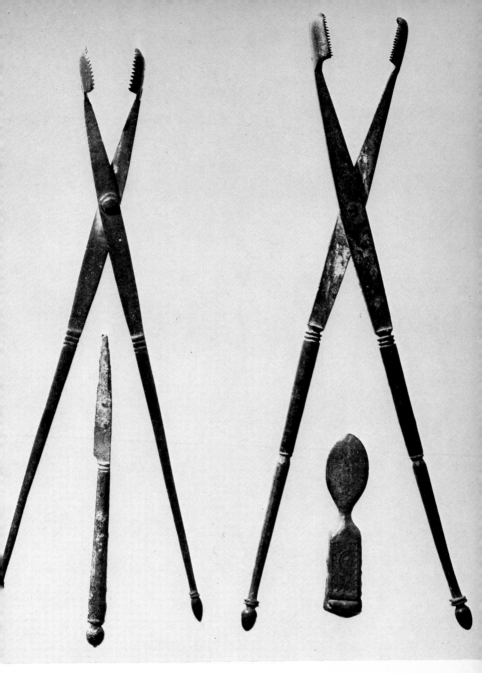

44 Two pairs of 'uvula' forceps; note the toothed grips; left, a narrow surgical knife probably used for cutting fine areas with the point; and, right, a short blunt probe. British Museum.

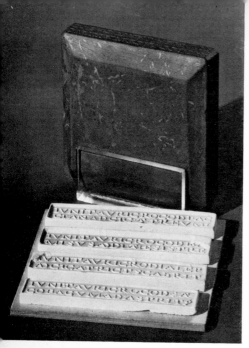
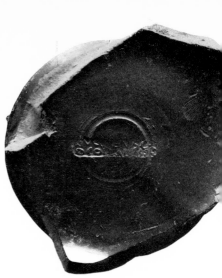

45–47 Eye diseases were among the most common complaints in the Roman Empire, usually treated by compounded salves. *Above, left,* an oculist's stamp of Junius Taurus from Naix (Meuse). It has prescriptions on all four edges; the upper one reads 'saffron ointment of Junius Taurus for scars and discharges; from the recipe of Paccius.' *Above, right,* the foot of a bowl from the City of London has a similar prescription for saffron ointment instead of the more usual potter's stamp (*C.I.L.* VII, 1314). *Below,* an oculist administers a salve to his patient's eye on a sarcophagus relief. British Museum and Ravenna.

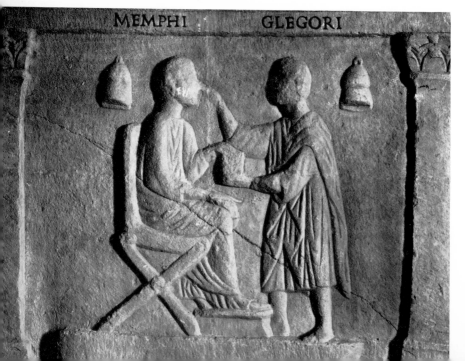

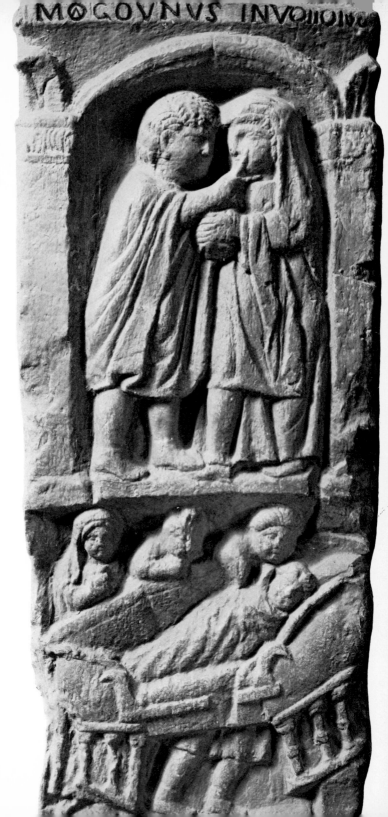

MOGOVNVS INVO...

This funerary
...e of a doctor,
...bably third–
...rth century AD,
...ws him in the
...per half
...mining a
...man's eye. The
...ne below, which
...curious
...spective, may
...resent the
...urners paying
...ir respects to
...deceased in his
...fin. Bar-le-Duc
...iseum.

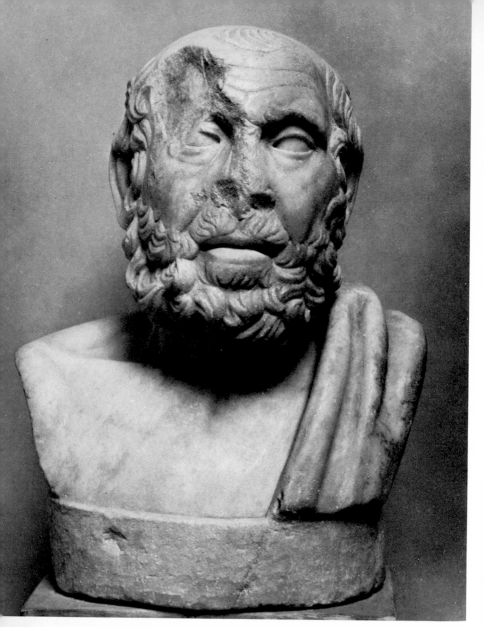

49 A Roman copy of a Hellenistic bust of Hippocrates. It was found at Ostia standing on a pedestal, bearing the Hippocratic Oath, before the tomb of K. Markios Demetrios. This portrait of the famous physician from Cos is probably one of the most authentic that we possess. Ostia Museum.

the achievement of Greek, Hellenistic, and Roman medicine. His work summarized all that was worthy in the medical traditions of the classical world, and until the rise of pre-Vesalian and Vesalian anatomy, or the development of chemistry and biophysics in the nineteenth and twentieth centuries, the Roman achievement withstood the test of centuries and remained the model upon which medical practice was built.

Cicero, Seneca, and many others summed the ideal of the physician as the Roman aristocrat perceived of him, and the social context imposed heavily, much as Morris and Sparks suggest for the origins of medical care. The Roman insisted his physician be a friend upon whom he could rely for solace when one of his illnesses appeared, or his valetudinarianism resulted in the matrix of the family, or he displayed self-assurance in medicine among his peers. The principles underlying medical care, suggested by Morris and his sources, give an excellent indication of the true achievement of Roman medicine: the recognition and treatment of those medical problems curable in the social context with a glimmer of objective observation of case histories and human and comparative anatomy. By modern standards, this medicine was severely limited, but it gave acceptable answers which were applied for 1,500 years, and provided the correct impetus and direction for the rise of modern medicine from Vesalius to Salk and de Bakey.

Proof of these concepts on the part of the educated in the Empire comes from many sources, but in particular from Plutarch's wide-ranging and discursive *Moralia*. He discusses just about everything that one pondered in the second century, and medicine and its related problems bulk large. Plutarch condemns superstition, as a rational Greek would normally do, simply because the 'superstitious man casts the doctor from his house', and 'classifies all diseases as afflictions of a god or attacks of an evil spirit.'[13] Plutarch does not deny that *some* diseases result from these causes, but rather that *most* diseases can be treated by the physician. Plutarch recalls the literary tradition equating Death and the doctor as brothers, but both are healing.[14] The physician has some understanding of the mystery of death but the Roman fully senses that the doctor can do only so much. What the physician can do appears in surgery and in post-operative care, which some patients did not want after an operation. Plutarch says such a patient bears the pain of treatment but does not wait for it to benefit.[15] The doctor in all of his work hopes to foster a growth of what is sound and thus to preserve it as long as possible,[16] but sometimes effects a cure without the patient's knowledge of the process.[17] Medicine clearly cures many illnesses, but has its boundaries, as Galen expresses it some years later. Plutarch's ideal doctors move in the social world of the second century with grace and dignity which merit approval. They observe and treat but are assured when they see fevers or diseases resulting from obvious causes. When they perceive medical problems that originate from obscure causes, or which grow gradually, the doctor faces them with resignation and fear rather than cure.[18] Plutarch's concept of medicine is one which recognizes that medicine soothes all of man's problems,[19] much as Propertius expresses it in one of his poems.[20] The good doctor prescribes kindly treatment whenever he can, and sleep and diet rather than strong drugs form the major elements of the advice of the physician.[21] Plutarch's physician understands the power of assurance and confidence in the face of the patient's fears and he treats according to rational principles as much as he can.

Plutarch, speaking as an educated man, often writes about the principles of medicine as they are elucidated in the classical tradition. Achilles 'knew medicine' simply because he perceived the difference between ordinary diseases and those resulting from unfamiliar causes.[22] Medicine grows from reason, Plutarch asserts, and man can control his life in as far as reason will allow. Hesiod 'knew medicine' as he pays great attention to the daily course of life and matters such as wine-mixing, the value of water, baths, women, the proper time for intercourse, and the way in which infants should sit.[23] Man can mould the most important aspects of his life according to this medical knowledge, which is a part of his intellectual heritage. Yet Plutarch goes further. He says everyone ought to know the peculiarities of his own pulse, because there are so many varieties, as well as the individual traits his own body has in temperature and dryness. Then one ought to be aware of what things in *actual practice* have proven to be beneficial or harmful to his own particular body-type.[24] The individual is responsible for knowing himself best and he should know what he digests best, or what (for him) constitutes a laxative or an agent of constipation, just as well as he knows what tastes sweet, bitter, and sour to him.[25] He should not bother the doctor with these questions as the physician has more important matters to attend to. Doctors treat fevers and toothaches, but sometimes patients reach a point in their diseases where they do not recognize the value of the doctor, in fact they do not realize they are ill. Frenzy and delirium prevent the doctor's care and the patient has recourse only to the kindness of his friends and the guarded hope of the doctor.[26] On the other hand, one's reason discerns between the ravings of a man who is very ill and a person who merely holds on to his injured member and screams (like little children). Here Plutarch borrows from Plato's *Republic*, and says, 'We ought to accustom our soul rapidly to the care of curing the wound and reassuring the fallen, and we ought to put aside sadness by the art of medicine.'[27] The concept is clear: medicine aids man's understanding of what he can do about physical ailments, and also points to the area in which his rational actions would be useful.

Plutarch's doctor possesses a certain level of technical skill. After surgery, the physician applies soothing lotions that are dependable.[28] The doctor ought to apply his medicines only after the body is unable to care for itself, and his skill is judged by his observation of the stages of inflammation and pain.[29] The physician knows his 'drug psychology' by making sure his medicaments smell like perfumes or have bright colours which do not repel patients.[30] None the less, the doctor has a sense of judgement, to know when the patient needs harsh drugs, such as polium, 'whose smell is awful', in preference to a bath or a generous diet. The doctor should be able to compound such as hellebore on the spot, and convince the patient of its worth in restoring health.[31] The physician uses his surgical tools to cure abscesses and tumours, but not to cut hair nor to trim fingernails.[32] A certain neatness and orderliness dominate the doctor's actions and the patient can judge his skill by the physician's assurance of his techniques in an operation.[33] He has good advice about diet, such as the general recommendation of allowing some time to intervene between dinner and sleep.[34] The doctor has read something of the earlier experiments, and can explain how blows to the left side of the body record the sensation on the right side.[35] He has some equipment with him, in addition to ordinary surgical implements, and has knowledge of the high repute of cupping glasses, discovered in Solon's day (so Plutarch says).[36]

Of course medicine leads to abuses. Drug dealers are not supposed to practise medicine, but they command a following much as the pseudo-philosophers who know just enough for display in the town square when the occasion arises.[37] Then, too, some patients take advantage of the physician's kindness and concern to remain rather shamefully in their beds for days. They receive many ointments and purges, and prove to be servile to the doctor, and they pay far too much attention to his talk. The doctor answers their silly requests for remedies to imaginary problems, and doses them with wine or cold water.[38] Plutarch condemns both physician and patient for warping the purpose of medicine, but we see the level of medicine enjoyed in the Empire by the educated. An Aristides based his search upon the concepts clarified by Plutarch, but found temporary help only in a personal relationship with a god.

Medical literature provides the counterpart for the effectiveness of Roman medicine to a given point. The doctor recognizes his limits, rather sadly, and offers what help he can. Aretaeus of Cappadocia, reputed as one of the best doctors of his day, states the problem with eloquence. He speaks of the treatment of tetanus.

> This is a misfortune which renders a man less than human. The sight of it is such as to fill one with a sense of hopelessness, and is one to fill the observer with great distress. It is a disease which is absolutely incurable. There is usually complete ignorance as to the cause of the change in the patient, even on the part of his dearest friends. At this point the prayer (which usually would not be fitting to the gods), that the victim be released from life, is a most fitting one, as it

would be a release from suffering and sorrowful evil in the patient's life. But a doctor, who is on the scene and observing, cannot help the patient preserve his life, nor can he give freedom from pain, nor can the physician alter the state of the patient. For if the doctor should wish to straighten out the patient's limbs, he can do so only by breaking or cutting in two the limbs of a living man. Thus the physician can offer only his sympathy to those who are overcome with this malady. This is a great misfortune for the doctor.[39]

Aretaeus recognizes the value of the positive approach to all patients, no matter what their complaints. Medical talent consists of perseverance, and how one varies treatment. The physician prescribes many pleasant and harmless things and gives encouragement whenever he feels the need to keep the patient in good spirits.[40] The patient has to possess a goodly amount of courage so that he can co-operate with the physician against the disease, but the physician should recognize that disease can take control of the body to the point of making the patient unaware of what he is saying or doing. The doctor thus should understand and know how he can help those whose diseases have not gained the upper hand, and observe those who have disorders of the senses, who may or may not recover health.[41] The attending physician can utilize many techniques and experiences to aid the sick, but once he has exhausted his stock of drugs, poultices, cupping glasses, theories of fluxes and their control through diet, the doctor simply says 'the patient cannot be cured.'[42] Shrewd judgement must form a major part of the physician's activities, and he should not administer drugs to a person on the verge of death from suffocation, since those observing might blame the doctor for the death of the patient. To Aretaeus the preservation of the physician's public image was most important. A doctor builds his repute on his timing of drug application and his judgement of whom to treat and whom to observe sadly.[43] Surgery aids the physician, although we look back and are somewhat thankful we do not have to undergo treatment for bladder stones from Celsus or Aretaeus.[44]
Celsus and Aretaeus display wide reading and experience in

medicine as it was known in the Roman Empire. Both have warmth and sympathy for their patients coupled with the kindly firmness necessary in successful surgery. Celsus emphasizes the need for careful observation of the sick man so that the doctor may prove his intellectual prowess by inventing new treatments if the disease is unknown.[45] Yet Celsus, as Galen, has an uneasy suspicion that matters which may not be understood cause illness.[46] Their consideration of 'hidden causes' and the earlier assertions of Erasistratus show the doctor trying to define what he can do. Celsus, like Aretaeus, admits that the physician must assume he cannot always give satisfactory answers.[47] Galen, also in reference to Erasistratus, admits the problem of recognition of disease, but inserts a dose of philosophico-medical jargon to side-step the question.[48] Again we are forced to face the riddle of why Galen and his colleagues found this dead-end in their practice for which they could offer no solution. Farrington's flat assertion of the 'horrible social reality' of slave labour in the classical world as the cause of limitations of ancient science[49] leaves the reader with the impression of a simplistic answer which fails to treat the roots of the classical mind. The demands on ancient medicine were more important, and Galen, Celsus, and the rest have a sublime mastery of illnesses which are soothed in the social context but which admit the limit of man's understanding. The age of unlimited belief in scientific answers was not at hand, and medicine was but a specialized segment of generalized concepts in philosophy and traditions, given organization and effectiveness by the spurt of Alexandria and the shift to encyclopedic collections of observations in the Empire. Galen's work stands as the culmination of these efforts. It is the most complete 'encyclopedia' of medicine in the classical world, and not much could be added to it until Vesalius.

Roman imperial society was a complex of many traditions, and none was stronger than religious medicine. The Hellenistic world bequeathed to the eastern half of the Empire a long history of famous medical shrines, and these centres grew in influence and exerted enormous authority, readily admitted by Galen.[50] The ordinary citizen observed medicine practised on many levels, particularly the lowest with its attendant fraud and quackery.

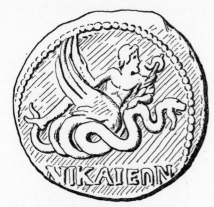

Fig. 15 Bronze medallion of Severus Alexander (AD 222–235) of Nicaia, Asia Minor. The reverse shows Asclepius riding a dragon (vide W. H. Waddington, Rec. Gen. Mon. Grec., pl. LXXXII, 24; diam. 1 in.)

Often his best recourse was to one of the medical shrines which enjoyed a favourable reputation among the masses. The sanctuaries to Asclepius dotted the Empire from Britain to Phoenicia and from the north shore of the Black Sea to Egypt, Africa, and Spain.[51] Evidence of cults of Asclepius loom large in our archaeological finds, and the legends of Asclepius the Healer spring from origins as old as Greek thought itself.[52] The citizen of the Empire had local access to this form of medical care and trusted it.

The modern reader should attempt to recall how important superstition (or what *we* call superstition) was to medicine in the Roman world, as he tries to understand how the Roman citizen found worth in the religious medical shrines scattered throughout his Empire. Pliny helps us as he writes of the natural and normal belief that medicine was a part of the world of nature, and had to be studied and approached as were all other phenomena from nature. There was a kind of sympathy and antipathy in all nature, and there were friendships and hostilities within everything that man could not speak to directly, that is the world possessing no soul. Since this was the pattern of nature, it followed that remedies for all ailments were common and easily discovered, and only man corrupted the order of things by his own greed and deception in making expensive rarities of medicines.[53]

Inscriptions occasionally provide glimpses of the men who felt the reality of the unseen, unfeeling world. The Roman citizen understood a deeper meaning to the cure from any of the shrines, at Pergamon or elsewhere, and the sacred symbols spoke of life at the threshold of death.[54] In the mind of the Roman or the Greek, it might appear as an unknown force, cold and without light, which could be warm and radiant, and which had a life of its own just beneath the surface of the real world. This force worked the cure and it was an exact experience, immediate in its communication, with the divine force in the natural miracle of the extension of life in the form of healing. The visit to Epidaurus or Pergamon was not a visit to a doctor's stall. The patient hoped to meet the naked and instant event of healing expressed to him in dreams and visions which took symbolic or real forms. Following long-accepted custom, he isolated himself from his fellows in the experience of healing and trusted his problem to the natural forces which he knew always to be a part of himself.[55] Votives measured only the results and were attempts to express the external awe at the miracle of religious experience.

Magic and religion were so intertwined as to be usually indistinguishable to the Roman and his subjects. Terracotta figurines from Egypt indicate the strength of magico-medical tradition.[56] The Tiber Island, so famous for its medical powers, had a complicated history of amalgam of many magical and medical traditions. According to the story, the god Vediovis as well as the Greek Apollo and Aesculapius, were fused in the traditional authority of the Tiber Island.[57] Pausanias records early traditions in Thessaly that indicated a long-lasting association of Apollo and Asclepius.[58] The shrines of Asclepius had healthful locations and springs of which Plutarch and Vitruvius speak with great enthusiasm.[59] Medical phenomena considered uncommon were given religious connotation as a matter of normal opinion.[60] Horace expresses it well:

The words of the wise on magic charms you can use
To soothe the pain and practically rout the disease.

Fig. 16 Detail from the plan of the temple and 'Long Building' at Lydney, Glos. It has been suggested that the 'Long Building', with its individual rooms, was used by the suppliant at the shrine seeking a cure via ritual incubation (or temple-sleep). (After R. E. M. Wheeler, Lydney, pl. LI)

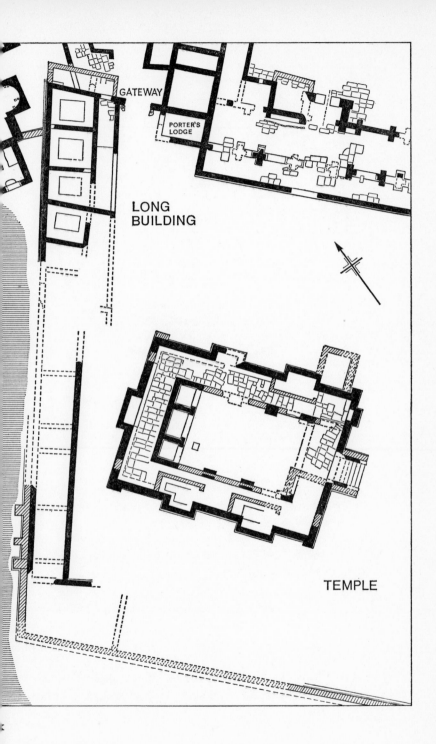

GATEWAY

PORTER'S
LODGE

LONG
BUILDING

TEMPLE

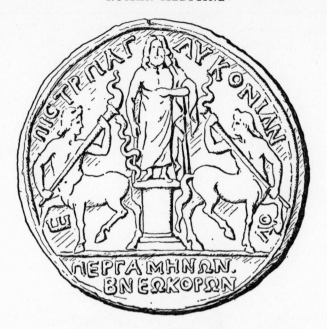

Fig. 17 Bronze medallion of Commodus (AD 180–192) of Pergamon, Asia Minor. The reverse shows the cult (?) statue of Asclepius on a plinth flanked by two backward-looking centaurs holding flaming torches (vide T. E. Mionnet, Descr. de Med.11. no. 200; diam. 1·6 in.)

Or is your tumour ambition? Miracle cures
In the booklet will renovate you: just read them through
Three times in the right frame of mind . . .[61]

Galen liked to have his patients think he possessed some sort of mysterious power in medicine, even though he explained (in his writing) his cure through rational means. Galen felt he had succeeded well when a patient departed in wonder at his powers.[62] Ulpian admonishes the general attitude by noting, 'those who chant, or those who expel evil spirits, should not be thought of as physicians.'[63]

In his remedy-book, Dioscorides includes instructions for men digging up hellebore. They should stand up and pray to Apollo and Aesculapius, and an eagle flying over their heads meant their death.[64] Libanius has his ills cured through magic and the ministrations of Asclepius, who appeared to him in three visions. His observations, like those of Aristides, are an excellent reflection of an age of visions, magic, and generally accepted unworldly matters.[65]

Of course, many intellectuals in the Roman world attacked superstition and its general acceptance. Cicero, Favorinus, Sextus Empiricus, and Lucian wrote treatises condemning the hope that astrology and magic can be used by man as tools to know the secrets of the unseen world. Roman practical logic refuted such knowledge on the ground that it would do man no good, and would tamper with forces which were to be respected, not seen or understood.[66] There are hints in Cicero and Lucian of the great contempt for the obvious belief of the masses in magic and astrology, and the disdain follows from the class structure in the Empire where 'the many' believe in magic but the sceptics at the top do not. Lucian denies magic not for reasons put forth in the modern world, but because there are matters man has no business investigating.

Within the question of understanding the Roman concept of himself and his relation to the world of nature, lies a deeper, and in some respects unsolvable, ambiguity of language. Whenever we attempt to render conceptualizations as expressed by Pliny or Galen into modern tongues, we overdefine and impose a modern clarity of concept which does little justice to the ancient view of medicine or nature. If the Romans thought in terms of 'science', they did so only with *scientia*, rather than a full-fledged distinction in areas of study. It is this problem which causes many a modern student of antiquity to assume his concepts of the normal were the concepts of the normal in the Roman world. He sometimes sees his hero(es) as a kind of stereotype fitting his own immediate impressions of what *should* be. Our first duty appears to be to recognize that differences exist between our own and the Roman conceptualization of the natural world. Hopkins states the problem well as he writes, 'if we can assume some harmony between conceptualization of total environment on the one hand and personality on the other, differences in conceptualization would

lead one to expect differences in personalities. . . . Human "nature"
if it is to be used at all [to explain history] may more reasonably be
seen as variable, not constant, and this degree of variability is a
proper subject for investigation not assumption.'[67] Thus the usual
approach of development-by-accumulation cannot answer questions about the methods pursued by Roman medicine. No so-
called scientific patterns directed efforts, but work rested on a set
of traditional approaches allowing the individual to interpret his
life in connection with the world in which he lived, not in isolation from it. This led to the incorporation of 'scientific' magic,
religion, and astrology, as well as a tradition of anatomy and
physiology, into Roman medical concepts. The doctor mastered
his craft with the knowledge that there were forces existing,
understood by respecting their very being, not by 'knowing' how
they worked.

Roman medicine was a summary of medical traditions from
the Greek, Hellenistic, and Roman worlds, and reflected a growing
tendency to incorporate more and more non-rational elements
into its thinking, as did Roman society as a whole by Galen's day.
Yet the irrational was always a major portion of the intellectual
world of antiquity, even the Greek mind at its best.[68] It should
come as no surprise to discover magic, superstition, and religion
as real forces to the individual in the Empire. Fear, however, is not
a designation appropriate to the view. Greek and Roman religion
existed through many centuries as an attempt at the definition by
man of his correct relation to the unknown or divine forces
motivating human existence and history.

As a part of the social and cultural heritage, Roman medicine
refined and improved it to a point where men were better able to
see the relationship in the classical definition. True, the pattern
came to include more physical manifestations, but for the Roman
the system of medicine answered cogent problems and performed
an effective task in its many roles. It is only when we, as members
of a later society, with the gifts of hindsight and differing ideals,
attempt to define Roman medicine in modern terms that it falls
short. One should recall the basic humanity of Celsus, Aretaeus,
and Galen as one assesses the worth of medicine in the Empire.

BIOGRAPHICAL SKETCHES

THE FOLLOWING are in no way intended to be exhaustive, but are provided to put the physicians and authors into historical context. For biographical details, see Sarton, *Introduction*, Diepgen, *Geschichte der Medizin*, I, the *Oxford Classical Dictionary*, and the various volumes of *PWK*. For the confused chronology of the Hellenistic physicians, Michler, *Die alexandrinischen Chirurgen*, 23–8, gives a good summary.

AELIUS ARISTIDES (118–89). A Sophist, educated at Pergamon and Athens. Widely travelled in Egypt and Asia Minor, arriving in Rome in 156. Not very effective as a teacher of rhetoric, but excelled in giving set speeches for various occasions. Fifty-five of these survive. Wrote the 'Sacred Discourses' as well as eulogies of Rome, Smyrna, and Athens, congratulations to the Emperor, and an attack on philosophy. Used Attic style. Good example of sophistic eloquence of the second century with rhetorical devices. Suffered his 'illnesses' off and on from 141 to 171. *Vid*. C. A. Behr, *Aelius Aristides* (Amsterdam, 1968).

AGATHINUS of Sparta (fl. 60–100). Regarded as the founder of Eclecticism. Wrote a short work on the pulse, and on the action of hellebore, based on experiment.

ANDREAS (d. 217 BC at the Battle of Raphia). Physician to Ptolemy IV. Wrote books on snakebite, a treatise against superstition, and a work considering descriptions of plants and animals.

ANDROMACHUS of Crete (fl. 54–68). Physician to Nero. Skilled in compounding drugs. Medical histories usually call him the 'Elder' to distinguish him from his son, also a physician and a drug-specialist.

ANTYLLUS (fl. c. 110–130). Famous as a skilled surgeon, and quoted through Archigenes by Galen. Fragments mostly in Oribasius. Antyllus made a study of venesection and cupping, and wrote down detailed instructions for operations (cataracts, tracheotomy).

APOLLONIUS MYS (fl. in Alexandria c. 30 BC). Wrote works *On the Herophileans*, *On Cheap Drugs*, and *On Unguents*.

ARCHAGATHUS of Sparta (?) (fl. in Rome c. 220 BC). Traditionally the first Greek physician to settle in Rome.

ARCHIGENES of Apamaea (Syria) (fl. in Rome c. 100–117). Pupil of Agathinus, from whom he got most of his medical theory. Archigenes taught elaborate pulse theory, and invented a classification of four stages of fever and four stages of disease.

ARETAEUS of Cappadocia (c. 120–180). Greek physician of Eclectic leanings, who espoused the Pneumatic school. Taught simple therapeutics, and recognized differences between cerebral and spinal paralysis. His work often reflected good sense at the expense of theory.

ASCLEPIADES of Bithynia (b. c. 120 BC in Prusa, fl. in Rome c. 90–75 BC). Hopeful teacher of rhetoric turned physician, settled in Rome and took up medicine as taught by Cleophantus and the atomistic school. Advocated mechanistic medicine which appealed to his Roman patients. Placed no value on the study of anatomy.

ATHENAEUS of Naucratis (Egypt) (fl. c. 200). Wrote the *Deipnosophistae* some time after the death of Commodus (192). The 'banquet' extends over several days, and the guests represent learned fields, in the manner of the Platonic symposium. The work is far inferior to Plato, but has enormous value for the excerpts of material, generally lost, which the guests recite from memory. Diphilus of Siphnos would otherwise be unknown, and the Middle and New Comedy provide examples which are found nowhere else.

ATHENAEUS of Attalia (fl. under Claudius (41–54) in Rome). Reputed founder of the Pneumatic sect. Borrowed from Stoics the ideas of the four elements, and added a fifth, the *pneuma*. Moods (as we define them) used for diagnosis: disease and health explained by their *eukrasia* (good temperament) or *dyskrasia* (bad temperament). Considered medicine part of general education. Galen thinks highly of Athenaeus.

BACCHIUS of Tanagra (fl. *c.* 200 BC). Herophilean who wrote a glossary on the works of Hippocrates. Famed for skilled prescription of drugs.

CAELIUS AURELIANUS (fl. *c.* 410?). Epitomizer and translator of Soranus' works, *Acute Diseases* and *Chronic Diseases*. Also translated a large portion of Soranus' *Gynaecia*. Important for the defence of the Methodistic methods against others, whose works are lost. Provides information on Diocles, Praxagoras, Asclepiades, Heracleides of Tarentum, Themison, and Thessalus. *Vid.* introduction to Drabkin's *Caelius Aurelianus: Acute Diseases and Chronic Diseases*.

CASSIUS the Sicilian (fl. in Rome *c.* 14–25). Obscure doctor chosen by M. Wellmann, *Celsus: eine Quellenuntersuchung* (Berlin, 1913) as the 'source' of Celsus' 'translation'.

MARCUS PORCIUS CATO, the Censor (Cato the Elder) (234–149 BC). Born of peasant ancestry in Tusculum. Served with distinction in the Second Punic War and was present at the Metaurus (207 BC). Lucius Valerius Flaccus recognized Cato's legal aptitude and started him along his *cursus honorum*. Quaestor (204 BC), brought Ennius to Rome (203 or 202 BC), Consul (195 BC), served with honour in the war against Antiochus III, Censor (184 BC). Wrote *On Agriculture c.* 160 BC. Other works (*Origines, Letters*, etc.) lost except for fragments.

AULUS (?) CORNELIUS CELSUS (fl. in Rome *c.* 14–37). Wrote an encyclopedia in Latin on rhetoric, philosophy, law, the military, and medicine. Only treatise on medicine survives. Theory and practice of medicine well knit into the Roman pragmatic approach, with strong tradition of family medicine. One of the basic sources (with Galen and Oribasius) for Hellenistic medicine. Valued by Columella and Quintilian. For unknown reasons, Celsus was lost during the Middle Ages, but was received with enthusiasm upon rediscovery in the early Renaissance (1426).

CHRYSIPPUS of Cnidus (fl. *c.* 370 BC). Physician associated with the traditions of the Cnidian centre of medical instruction. Wrote a treatise on vegetables, noting the health-promoting properties of cabbage. Follower of Eudoxus and Philistion.

CLEOPHANTUS (fl. *c.* 160 BC at Alexandria [?]). Erasistratean surgeon and gynaecologist. Traditionally the medical inspiration for Asclepiades of Bithynia.

LUCIUS JUNIUS MODERATUS COLUMELLA (*c.* 10–*c.* 70). Spaniard from Gades, served as tribune in the Legio VI Ferrata in Syria and Cilicia (*c.* 36. *CIL*, IX, 235). Wrote his *On Agriculture c.* 60. His *On Trees* survives, but his *Against the Astrologers* and *On the Rites of Purification* are lost. Style clear, with major inspiration from Vergil's *Georgics*.

DEMETRIUS of Apamaea (Syria) (fl. 110–90 BC). Specialist in gynaecology and obstetrics. Known only through fragments in Soranus and Caelius Aurelianus.

DEMOCEDES of Crotona (b. at Crotona, fl. at Athens, Aegina, Samos, and at the court of Darius 521–485 BC). Presumably died at Crotona. Had Pythagorean system of medicine. Story of his cure for the Persian queen is in Herodotus, III, 129–38.

DIOCLES of Carystos (Euboea) (fl. c. 360–330 BC). Synthesizer of Sicilian and Coan approaches to medicine. Called by the Athenians a 'second Hippocrates'. First doctor to write in Attic, and known to carry out experiments in dissection. Wrote on medical botany and was source for Theophrastus.

DIOSCORIDES (fl. c. 41–68 in Rome). Wrote a compendium of all the materia medica then known from Greek medicine and other sources. May have learned his medicine by practical experience while in the legions. His work describes some 600 plants and their possible medical use.

DIPHILUS of Siphnos (fl. c. 305–280 BC under King Lysimachus). Wrote books on diets. Fragments extant only in Athenaeus' *Deipnosophistae*.

ERASISTRATUS of Iulis (Ceos, the Cyclades) (b. c. 304 BC and fl. in Alexandria c. 260 BC). Younger contemporary of Herophilus, borrowed his medical ideas from the Dogmatic school of Praxagoras. Great physiologist. Came close to discovering circulation. Recognized every organ had arteries, veins, and nerves.

EUDEMUS of Alexandria (fl. c. 240 BC). Anatomist, younger contemporary of Erasistratus. Studied the nervous system, human osteology, female sex organs, and experimented in embryological studies.

EVENOR of Argos (fl. c. 380 BC in Athens). A gynaecologist and ophthalmologist of repute. Usually labelled Dogmatic. Noted for his introduction of speculation into the Hippocratic method. Wrote a book *On Treatments*.

SEXTUS JULIUS FRONTINUS (*c.* 30–104). Praetor Urbanus (70), *consul suffectus* (73), governor of Britain (74–78). Was *curator aquarum* under Trajan, and wrote *On Aqueducts* while in this position. Also wrote *Stratagems*, which survives (Book IV may be spurious), and treatises on military matters and surveying which do not.

MARCUS CORNELIUS FRONTO (*c.* 100–*c.* 166; b. at Cirta, Numidia). Most noted orator of his day. *Cursus honorum* recorded in *CIL*, VIII, 5350. *Consul suffectus* in 143. Was tutor for the future emperors Marcus Aurelius and Lucius Verus. His *Correspondence* discovered in Milan (by Mai) in 1815 as palimpsest.

GALEN of Pergamon (*c.* 129–200). Studied medicine at Pergamon, Smyrna, Corinth, and Alexandria. Functioned as gladiatorial doctor at Pergamon, 157–161. First sojourn in Rome, 162–166. Summoned by Marcus Aurelius in 169. Galen became physician to the heir-apparent Commodus after 169. Probably died in Rome. Prolific writer and compiler, not a great mind, but had ability of synthesis. His work forms the greatest corpus of material we possess of classical medicine.

AULUS GELLIUS (*c.* 123–*c.* 165; b. in Rome). Studied literature, and was a good friend of Fronto. Visited Athens, later functioned as judge in private cases in Rome. Wrote *Attic Nights* as a collection of various tidbits of law, grammar, history. Probably published under Marcus Aurelius. *Attic Nights* is a good example of archaism in the Roman literature of the second century.

GLAUCIAS of Tarentum (fl. *c.* 70 BC). Tarentine physician, wrote treatises on medical herbs and lexicon of Hippocrates.

HERACLEIDES of Tarentum (fl. *c.* 70 BC). Pupil of Mantias, the most famous of the 'Empirical' physicians of his day. Made experiments on the properties of opium.

HERODOTUS (fl. in Rome *c.* 70–100). Pupil of Agathinus, with leanings towards Methodism, showing the outlook of the Eclectics. His fragments exist mainly in Oribasius.

HEROPHILUS of Chalcedon (fl. at Alexandria *c.* 300 BC). Best anatomist in the Hellenistic tradition. Conducted many original dissections in the Alexandrian Museum, and was first to do systematic work on the human body.

HICESIUS of Smyrna (fl. *c.* 60 BC). Wrote much on drugs and diet. Noted for a special plaster.

HIPPOCRATES of Cos (*c.* 460–*c.* 380/370 BC). Most famous physician of antiquity. The medical writings of the Coan centre came to be associated with his name. A basic rationalism of disease is his major contribution.

LYCUS of Macedonia (d. *c.* 170). Pupil of Quintus, classed as an Empiric. Especially disliked by Galen. Wrote books on muscles, in which he omitted the pterygoid and various neck muscles. No work survives. Galen, XVIII, 1, 196–245 (*Adversus Lycum*) seems to show why.

MANTIAS (fl. 110 BC). Herophilean doctor whose main claim to repute was that he had taught Heracleides of Tarentum.

MARCELLUS EMPIRICUS of Bordeaux (fl. 310–410). Gallo-Roman physician, *magister officiorum* under Theodosius I (379–395). Wrote his book of medicaments *c.* 410, which shows impact of superstition and Celtic popular remedies.

MARINUS (fl. *c.* 130). Anatomist, often mentioned by Galen. Probably lived at Alexandria. Wrote works on the roots of nerves, muscles, commentary on Aphorisms, as well as books on anatomy.

MENODORUS (fl. *c.* 60 BC). Friend of Hicesius (Athenaeus, II, 59). Wrote drug recipes and some works on wounds of the head.

MOLPIS (fl. *c.* 175 BC [?]). Famous for his techniques of relief for dislocations.

NILEUS (fl. *c.* 200 BC). Herophilean physician, praised by Celsus, VIII, 20. 4, as one of his most eminent authorities. Famous for his operative technique in ophthalmology.

NUMESIANUS (fl. *c.* 150). Anatomist and exponent of Hippocrates. Classed as Dogmatic. Taught anatomy to Galen and Pelops.

NYMPHODORUS (fl. *c.* 200 BC [?]). Noted for his combination of surgery with a use of drugs.

ONASANDER (fl. *c.* 49–59). Antiquarian. Wrote a treatise on the duties and qualities of a military commander ('On Strategy') *c.* 49. No claim to originality, but shows something of the Hellenistic military tradition as the early Roman Empire remembered it.

ORIBASIUS (*c.* 325–*c.* 400). Greek encyclopedist-physician. Borrowed heavily from Galen, and helped prepare the way for Galen's later popularity among Byzantines and Arabs. Friend and physician to the Emperor Julian (361–363). Wrote huge medical encyclopaedia in 70 books, of which a third survives. His compendium fundamental for our knowledge of earlier medical authorities as he quotes them carefully and meticulously.

PELAGONIUS (fl. *c.* 365). Writer on veterinary medicine, a compilation of many sources (Greek) but also from Columella and Celsus. Used by Vegetius.

PELOPS (fl. *c.* 155). Classed as a Dogmatist. Exponent of humoral pathology. Wrote books on anatomy, which were burned. Held that arteries, nerves, veins, all rise in the brain.

PHILISTION of Locri (*c.* 427–347 BC). A representative of the Sicilian school of medicine. From Empedocles, assumed four elements (fire, air, water, earth) which he equated with hot, cold, moist, dry, in turn responsible for all body functions. His *On Dietetics* famous in antiquity.

PHILOTIMUS (fl. *c.* 315 BC). Wrote on pleurisy and epilepsy. Caelius Aurelianus, *Chronic Diseases*, I, 4. 140, derides him for his errors.

PHILOXENUS (fl. *c.* 75-50 BC). Called Claudius Philoxenus by Galen (XIII, 539, 645); a surgeon of Alexandrian training.

GAIUS PLINIUS SECUNDUS (Pliny the Elder) (23-79). Born at Comum, to Rome as a youth for his education. Served in cavalry in Germany, and was procurator (in succession) of Gallia Narbonensis, Africa, Hispania Tarraconensis, and Gallia Belgica under Vespasian. His last post was admiral of the fleet at Misenum, and he died from fumes while sailing for a closer look at the eruption of Vesuvius, August 24, 79. His *Natural History* dedicated to Titus in 77. Other works such as *On the Javelin in Cavalry*, the *German Wars* (used by Tacitus) and the rest lost. Exhibits enormous energy, uncritical use of sources, goodnatured love of the extraordinary, omnivorous appetite for antiquarian minutiae. The *Natural History* is a mine for such varied matters as the histories of sculpture, art, folklore, and medicine, while being an encyclopedia of life and customs of the Roman world in the first century.

PLUTARCH of Chaeronea (*c.* 46-127). Son of an Academic philosopher and biographer. In the 60's studied physics, natural science and rhetoric at Athens. Visited Rome, was friend of the philosopher, Favorinus. Great enthusiasm for ethics. Welltravelled over the east, and had a private school at Chaeronea. Was a priest of Delphi after 95. Wrote *Moralia* and parallel *Lives*, which remain popular. First goal political and moral virtues, not history. Habit of anecdote makes Plutarch's work rich in varia on many topics.

PRAXAGORAS of Cos (fl. 320–280 BC). The most famous physician, after Diocles, in the Dogmatic tradition. The first to draw a distinction between veins and arteries (arteries carry air; veins carry blood), and did further work on theories of the pulse.

PROTARCHUS (fl. c. 150 BC [?]). Surgeon, noted for his combination of mechanical knowledge with pharmacology.

QUINTUS (fl. c. 120). Teacher of Satyrus and Numesianus. Expelled from Rome for unknown reasons.

QUINTUS SMYRNAEUS (fl. c. 350). Poet with aspirations for epic. Wrote *The Fall of Troy* to continue the *Iliad* to the start of the homeward journey of the Achaeans (hence, called sometimes the *Posthomerica*).

RUFUS of Ephesus (c. 110–c. 180 in Rome and Egypt). Good anatomist, described optic chiasma, wrote a work on the pulse which may show he understood difference between diastole and systole. Based his work on Herophilus, but did more detailed work on monkeys and pigs.

SATYRUS of Pergamon (fl. c. 150). Galen's first teacher of anatomy. Wrote commentaries on Hippocrates which are lost. Probably the same Satyrus who tried to give Aelius Aristides sensible advice.

SCRIBONIUS LARGUS (fl. c. 14–54 in Rome). Pharmacologist who published in Latin his *Compositiones medicamentorum*, c. 47. Shows folk origins and influence of magic.

SERAPION of Alexandria (c. 200–150 BC). Reputed founder of the Empirical school. Placed individual observation first, opinions of authorities second, and analogy third. Galen has high praise for him.

QUINTUS SERENUS SAMMONICUS (fl. under Septimius Severus). Killed by Caracalla *if* he is the same Serenus Sammonicus of *SHA, Caracalla*, IV, 4. Famous as collector of books (supposedly had 62,000 vols; *SHA, The Three Gordians*, XVIII, 2–3) and known for his knowledge of poetic speeches (*SHA, Severus Alexander*, XXX, 2). Probably is the author of *Liber medicinalis*. Important for Roman medical concepts as he cites Plautus (XXII, 24 [425]), Lucretius (XXXII, 4 [606]), Horace (XXVII, 16–17 [528–529]) as medical authorities, along with Varro and Pliny. Arrangement of the work much like Scribonius Largus with much magic.

SILIUS ITALICUS (Tiberius Catius Asconius Silius Italicus) (*c.* 26–*c.* 101). Wrote the *Punica* after 88. Borrows from Livy, Varro, Hyginus, Posidonius, Valerius Antias, Lucan, but owes greatest debt to Vergil. *Punica* longest Latin poem, historical epic on the Second Punic War. Gruesome battle descriptions.

SORANUS of Ephesus (fl. *c.* 98–138 in Rome). Finest example of the Methodist tradition, and one of the best gynaecologists of antiquity. *Vid.* introduction to Temkin's *Soranus' Gynecology*.

PUBLIUS PAPINIUS STATIUS (*c.* 45–96). Poet. Son of schoolmaster of Naples. Wrote the *Thebais* (pub. *c.* 91) and *Silvae* (92–96: the fifth published posthumously), the latter commemorating various ordinary topics, illuminating the life of the Roman country gentleman at the end of the first century.

THEMISON of Laodicaea (fl. *c.* 50 BC). Pupil of Asclepiades, reputed as the founder of the Methodist outlook. Taught the use of leeches in bleeding, and experimented with drugs.

THEODORUS PRISCIANUS. Served the emperor Gratian (367–383) as physician. Wrote a book of medicine, the *Euphoriston* or *Medicinae praesentae*, a collection of prescriptions. *Vid.* German translation in T. Meyer, *Theodorus Priscianus und die römische Medizin* (Jena, 1909; rpt. Wiesbaden, 1967).

THEOPHRASTUS of Eresos (Lesbos) (*c.* 372–*c.* 288 BC). Pupil of Aristotle, succeeded his teacher as head of the Lyceum (323–*c.* 288 BC). One of the great botanists of antiquity, the first to use the expanded data gained from Alexander's conquests. Two of his botanical works survive, and his treatise *On Stones* has recently been edited and translated by D. E. Eichholz (Oxford, 1965). Theophrastus taught that intellect had its seat in the brain, contradicting Aristotle who thought the heart was the centre of human intelligence. Theophrastus' works became culling grounds for authorities after him. Enormous influence.

THESSALUS of Tralles (Caria) (fl. *c.* 70–95 in Rome). Greek physician of Methodistic outlook. Took as his model Themison, and taught that all medicine was a result of clinical experience and teaching.

MARCUS TERENTIUS VARRO (116–27 BC). Born in Sabine country and later a pupil of the first known Roman philologist (Lucius Aelius Stilo). Fought with the Pompeians, but Caesar pardoned him, appointing him as curator of the future public library (47 BC). Wrote his *Rerum rusticarum* in 37 BC with emphasis on veterinary medicine on the Roman farm. His *De lingua latina* (pub. 43 BC) survives as Books V and VI of the whole, with pieces of Books VII–X. Encyclopedist who incorporated the Roman spirit of application into his work.

FLAVIUS VEGETIUS RENATUS (fl. *c.* 385). Wrote treatises, *Mulomedicina* and *Epitoma rei militaris*. Both appear as second-hand guidebooks. *Mulomedicina* uses Columella, Pelagonius, and a vulgar Latin version of a Greek *Hippiatrika*. The military handbook is an arrangement of literary materials from Cato to his own day.

VITRUVIUS POLLIO. Roman architect and military engineer under Augustus. Wrote *On Architecture*, considering architecture and engineering, from his own experience and like works by Hermogenes and other Greek architects. Hellenistic mood permeates the whole.

XENOCRATES (fl. *c.* 70 in Rome). Wrote books on drugs full of magic and superstition, as well as a treatise *On the Meaning of the Flight of Birds*. One of the sources of Pliny's *Natural History*.

ZEUXIS of Tarentum (fl. *c.* 60 BC). Independent-minded Herophilean. Founded centre for medical studies at Laodicaea in Syria.

SOURCES AND PROBLEMS

THE CONSIDERATION of Roman medicine is riddled with problems, many relating to the consideration of our sources. Archaeology helps to confuse more often than it clarifies, and the literary remains of the great medical treatises of the Empire suffer from mutilation and the bias of self-justification. One fact emerges from all points of evidence: the Romans did consider medicine important enough to discuss it and to consider its various aspects, but we must be extremely cautious in how we treat the regard.

Archaeological evidence consists of tools, presumably used in medical pursuits, as well as coins on occasion, inscriptions, the remains of structures (the *valetudinaria* of the legionary *castra*, or the so-called 'House of the Surgeon' in Pompeii), and the numerous remnants from the many Asclepia in the Empire. Problems arise as we attempt to assess the value of these fragments, tantalizing and tempting as many of them prove to be. For many of them, unless we chance to find literary references to identify individual or artistic styles of tools and the like, there is no automatic dating process, even when coins turn up in a dig. Coins tend to be hoarded, and we are often confronted with a choice of a 'date' from many possibilities.[1] Then, too, most finds are by simple chance, unlike Pompeii, which allows us to pose some conclusions on historic context, and most finds out of context may not represent ordinary patterns of life or of medical practice. Or to put it another way, there is no assurance that a selection of surgical tools, finely produced, indicates a skilled surgeon in action, but rather we can conclude the Romans possessed a high skill in the technology of implement production—and that is all we can say for sure. Archaeology cannot tell us how the tools were used, unless we find support from literary evidence, and we interpret Galen or Celsus correctly. Were the scalpels and such used as we use them? Or did the ancients have other purposes in mind? The usual assumption brings modern use into full play, but there is grave danger in supposing similar intent within varying intellectual matrices. Archaeology can aid immeasurably by indicating the differences of the past from the present, and thus our views remain in the realm of educated conjecture, with the ever-present possibility of new evidence changing our guess.

The literary remains pose enigmas which appear to be clear at first glance. If we assume the specialized, fragmentary pattern of medicine as it has existed since the sixteenth century, and particularly since the middle of the nineteenth, we can interpret Greco-Roman medicine in our own terms, as has so often been done. On the other hand, if we investigate the questions before us, and attempt to beware of preconceived notions, we arrive at 'philosophy' before we see medicine. The background of Hippocratic medicine as it descends into the Hellenistic and Roman worlds gives certain general principles which mark it as one of the great achievements of the Greek mind. The basic breakthrough was the rationalization of disease, but Hippocratic medicine had little use for surgery or the study of anatomy as we conceive of it today (or even as Erasistratus and Herophilus used it), and, furthermore, stated baldly the general mistrust of drugs. Medicine existed (and our evidence is firm here) as a 'skill' practised as were the 'skills' of armour-making or pottery manufacture, and the 'skill' of gymnastics allied itself with medicine as seemed natural. In the Hellenistic world, many 'universal men' (sophists) taught that men could know almost anything, provided their minds were sharp enough to comprehend the subtleties of clever argument. Medicine was theoretical, much as Plato built his balanced ideal on what should be true, using the intellect as the major tool. The Alexandrian Museum flourished for only a short time, and the work of Herophilus and Erasistratus represented the exception which foreshadowed its early extinction. Medical teaching formed in the homes of those who espoused given manners of looking at medicine, and labels attached to groups of doctors (the so-called 'schools') reflected only what their teachers thought. Medicine and its terminologies were couched in philosophy, even as the curiosity of an Erasistratus tinkered with body functions.

When we turn to the medical sources themselves, we find Galen dominating, with his huge corpus summarizing all of the speculation and work which had preceded him. Other writings which have managed to survive, as Celsus, Rufus of Ephesus, Aretaeus of Cappadocia, Soranus and his epitomizer and translator Caelius Aurelianus, as well as lesser remains from such as Herodotus, Archigenes, and the rest, bear out the generalized conclusion of medical 'philosophy' as a learned skill in the Roman Empire. Celsus shows the Roman adaptive genius at work; his medicine proves sensible and down to earth, and he rejects much of the prolixity characteristic of the Hellenistic handbooks he probably consulted in organizing his masterly *On Medicine*. Cato, Varro, Vitruvius, Columella, and Pliny the Elder provide glimpses of the Roman confidence in dealing with medical problems in a non-technical way. Other literary references are numerous and scattered throughout Greek and Latin writing of the Empire, and most express scepticism for the professional physician, as they might for a practising sophist. Rarest of literary remains are the papyri which have no personal axes to grind, but those we do have again show the prominence of individual solutions in the form of magic, religious medicine, and the like. Private rancour colours many of the notices we have on doctors in the Empire, and we must use care with such writers as Tacitus and Cicero, as we do for Galen and others on the opposite side of the question. Philosophical medicine reached few in the Empire, the few able to understand the esoteric knowledge of the intellectual physician.

Unlike most of classical literature, medical writers have not experienced the profusion of translation and commentary characteristic of poets and historians in the Empire. Thus in more than one sense, we stand at the beginning of a period when the study of these authors will begin to receive its just due from classicists and philologists who may (hopefully) want to break new paths. Celsus can be found in a relatively good translation by W. G. Spencer in the Loeb Library, based on the painstaking work of

Marx. Secondary literature on Celsus is plentiful, but most of it fails to deal with linguistic problems and their interpretation in the study of Roman medicine. The bulk of Pliny's *Natural History* seems to discourage a detailed commentary, although some parts of this most important Roman pot-pourri have received meticulous attention (folklore). Pliny has been translated a number of times, with the most readily available being the ten volumes of the Loeb Library. Varro, Columella, Vitruvius, and Cato are also in the Loeb Library.

Galen forms the greatest corpus of information for Roman medicine, but except for isolated volumes of the *Corpus medicorum Graecorum*, no textual studies have been made. The monstrous (twenty volumes in twenty-two) Kühn edition of Galen is based upon Renaissance collative work, and many spurious works seem to be included. Apparently, modern translators have been hesitant to put Galen before the modern reader because of the widespread assumption of Kühn's unreliability. The fear of the text being so corrupt as to prohibit translation or commentary is largely unfounded.[2] The secondary literature on Galen in modern European languages is enormous, as indicated by K. Schubring's forty-four pages of listings—of merely the most important work—in volume XX of the reprint of Kühn's Galen (Hildesheim, 1965), but most efforts seek to elucidate one or another of Galen's experiments or points of brilliance, rather than putting him into context.[3] English translations of Galen are strangely limited. The Loeb Library has but one volume of Galen (*On the Natural Faculties*) which shows Galen at his best. Sarton, *Galen*, 101–7, lists (to 1954) the Galen available in English, and the list is amazingly short considering the bulk of Galen in Kühn. Since 1954, the following have appeared, which may give the interested reader, unversed in the classical tongues, other tastes of Galen. P. W. Harkins, trans., *Galen On the Passions and Errors of the Soul* (Columbus, Ohio, 1963); J. S. Kieffer, trans., Galen's *Institutio Logica* (Baltimore, 1964); C. Singer, trans., *Galen On Anatomical Procedures* (Oxford, 1956), and W. L. H. Duckworth, trans., *Galen On Anatomical Procedures: The Later Books* (Cambridge, 1962); C. M. Goss, '(Galen) On the Anatomy of the Uterus', *Anat. Rec.*, CXLIV (1962), 77–84; C. M.

Goss, '(Galen) On the Anatomy of Muscles for Beginners', *ibid.*, CXLV (1963), 477–502; C. M. Goss, '(Galen) On Anatomy of Nerves', *American Journal of Anatomy*, XVIII (1966), 327–36; and M. T. May, trans., *Galen On the Usefulness of the Parts of the Body* (Ithaca, New York, 1968), 2 vols.[4]

Galen is at once our most complete and our most difficult source for Roman medicine. He appears full of self-contradictions as he wrestles with the tradition of philosophical, speculative medicine bequeathed him and attempts to verify what he reads and hears. His anatomy is good as far as he is able to use analogies from monkeys and other animals to give man's structures, but he continually faces the insuperable problem of terminology. His natural arrogance, as a learned Greek among dolts, warps his common sense as he speaks of patients, but his probing revives—again for a very short time—actual dissection as had been advocated by the best of the Ptolemaic Museum. None the less, we should not be misled into believing that *all* good physicians procured animals for comparative dissection or vivisection. Galen put out his numerous 'guidebooks' as an answer to the lack of such work, and the expected happened: people took him at his word, as we can see with Oribasius and later Byzantine medicine. Galen combines his acute observation with astrology and magic and occasional bombastics, and most particularly with a sheer prodigiousness of writing, for which he became well-known in his own time.[5] Galen gives us most of our extant fragments of earlier physicians' writings, and blends them all into his system of medicine. The Roman Empire of the second century is the dominant theme, with its changing emphasis from the speculative to the accepted. It is for this basic reason we need to remember Galen as a Roman philosopher-physician, rather than a doctor who 'looked ahead of his time'.

The English reader may appreciate notices of what other medical authors are available to him. F. Adams, ed. and trans., *The Extant Works of Aretaeus, the Cappadocian* (London, 1856) and *The Seven Books of Paulus Aegineta* (London, 1844–47), renders a remarkable translation of both authors, although now somewhat outdated. His notes to *Paulus* are a mine of information. O.

Temkin, trans., *Soranus' Gynecology* (Baltimore, 1956), is excellent, with a good introduction, though with a rather narrow medical cast in some of the remarks. I. E. Drabkin, ed. and trans., *Caelius Aurelianus On Acute Diseases and On Chronic Diseases* (Chicago, 1950), is a fine translation with a good critical historical introduction. A. J. Brock's *Greek Medicine* (London, 1929), gives some selections from Rufus of Ephesus (112–29) as well as some further translations from Galen (130–246). J. V. Ricci, trans., *Aetios of Amida* (Philadelphia, 1950), suffers from being a translation of a sixteenth-century Latin translation (Janus Cornarius, Basle, 1542). R. T. Gunther, ed., *The Greek Herbal of Dioscorides* (rpt., New York, 1959), is but a re-editing of the seventeenth-century (1655) translation of John Goodyer.

ON HUMAN DISSECTION IN ROMAN MEDICINE

ALTHOUGH THERE IS LITTLE DOUBT that dissection was employed by the best physicians in antiquity for practical knowledge of internal structures, proof for human dissection—with the exception of Hellenistic Alexandria—is vague. Galen's *On Anatomical Procedures* shows a tradition of dissection (Galen, II, 220, in particular) which continued in the Roman Empire, and he seems to say human dissection was still practised in Alexandria. He writes that students should go to Alexandria for such study, but he emphasizes that his students will be especially pleased in finding actual human skeletons there. Does this indicate continued dissection? It would seem not, although the skeletons indicate that some human material was still in use for teaching purposes. Rufus of Ephesus (134) notes that one must dissect animals to learn something of internal structure, and sadly muses that formerly (apparently Alexandria) such learning came from human cadavers. Celsus often indicates that dissection is necessary for the physician (*Prooemium*, 40–2, 74) and human dissection is clearly indicated. Cicero notes dissection is usual for the best doctors (*Academica*, II, 122), and that there is no objection to the practice on a dead body (*Tusculan Disputations*, I, 43. 104). Yet Celsus says one can learn a great deal in chance observation from the wounds of soldiers or gladiators (*Prooemium*, 43) and seems to indicate that dissection of the human cadaver is not an absolute necessity. Celsus' medicine may be learned without dissection, although it proves to be necessary to the best physicians. Rufus shows that the study of medicine began with terminology, that is one learned the names of the various parts of the body, and the exercise had become formalized without dissection (Rufus, 133–4).

On the other hand, the custom of dissection—or vivisection—of human beings remains a moot point owing to the nature of our evidence. Celsus tells the well-known story of human vivisection at Alexandria by Herophilus and Erasistratus (*Prooemium*, 23–7). The tale is repeated by Tertullian (AD 155–222), *De anima*, 10 and 25, but the language is quite ambiguous. After calling Herophilus a butcher (*lanius*) in chapter 10, Tertullian rebukes Herophilus in chapter 25 for the use of an instrument in embryotomy, implying that both the embryos and the 'adults also dissected' were alive. The problem of human vivisection, or dissection, at Alexandria, is complicated by the silence of Galen, who hints that Erasistratus had not dissected either living animals or humans (Galen, V, 602–3). The traditional accounts of dissection and vivisection at Alexandria probably reflect the general disgust it engendered among observers, and the physicians there presumably indulged in dissection when they had a chance. Otherwise it becomes difficult to explain the monumental discoveries attributed to Erasistratus and Herophilus. The practice of vivisection presents more of a complex problem. Possibly contemporaries confused the dissection of the dead with that of the living since they disapproved the practice altogether. Africa, *Science*, 52, L. Edelstein, 'The Development of Greek Anatomy', *BHM*, III (1935), 235–48 (238 and 246), and I. E. Drabkin, 'On Medical Education in Greece and Rome', *BHM*, XV (1944), 333–51 (340), accept the stories of vivisection as valid. Africa remarks, 'Comparable abuse in modern times adds weight to the probability of cruel practices in Alexandrian medicine.' *Cf.* L. Edelstein, 'Die Geschichte der Sektion in der Antike', *QS*, III (1932), 100–56.

Galen's knowledge of human anatomy is quite good, leading one to suspect he had some experience with cadaver dissection, although he discreetly leaves such implications out of his writing. Galen, III, 423, seems to contain a statement which might indicate he had dissected humans, but the context leaves the reader in doubt as to whether Galen is explaining a parallel structure for humans from his dissections of animals, or the actual description from human dissection. Galen does tell us about his practice at the gladiatorial school at Pergamon (Galen, VI, 529; XIII, 564, 600–1; XVIII, 2, 567) and he observed a few structures in the torn bodies of his patients. Perhaps this is all the 'dissection' Galen experienced of the human body, but the question must remain in the realm of conjecture, owing to the prejudice of our sources and the ambiguity of terminology. *Cf.* remarks in M. T. May, 'Galen on Human Dissection', *JHM*, XIII (1958), 409–10.

SOME NOTES ON ROMAN VETERINARY MEDICINE

ALTHOUGH VETERINARY MEDICINE is strictly outside the study of medicine in itself, the Roman attitudes on the care of their animals are revealing in connection with their general opinions of medicine as a whole. As might be expected, the writers on agriculture are rich in advice on care and treatment of stock, and Varro explains how an ordinary farmer can treat most diseases of both men and animals from the principles he has gleaned on the farm (Varro, II, 5. 11). Pliny (VIII, 41. 97) notes that animals have the ability to lead men to cures useful for themselves, and he writes on care of dogs (VIII, 63. 152-3), and how the horse 'suffers from the same maladies as man' (VIII, 67. 166). Cato, Varro, Columella, Celsus, Gargilius Martialis, and Palladius prove that the Romans evolved from their farm experience a remarkable tradition of medical knowledge applicable to their animals of all types. In fact, Latin treatises on veterinary medicine were translated into Greek (Pelagonius), showing Roman dominance in this, a most practical undertaking.

It seems that the Roman army had special provision for its sick horses, at least in the later period (Hyginus, *Liber de munitionibus castrorum*, XXI, 22), which may have a parallel development to the famous *valetudinaria*. Vegetius, the author of the garbled military handbook mentioned in chapters V and VI above, is also the probable author of a rather well-written and carefully-organized manual on diseases of mules and horses (*Mulomedicina*) which is based on Pelagonius. Gargilius Martialis wrote a work on the treatment of diseases in cattle, a remnant of which, titled *ex corpore Gargili Martialis*, is found at the end of E. Lommatzsch's edition of Vegetius' *Mulomedicina* (Teubner, 1903). Pelagonius and Vegetius are the first specialized works on veterinary medicine which have come down to us, and both are a blending of the Roman farm tradition with the Greek *Hippiatrika*. (Text for the Greek veterinary background is E. Oder and C. Hoppe, *Corpus Hippiatricorum Graecorum* (Teubner, 1924–27), and the Latin translation of the *Hippiatrika* is edited by E. Oder (Teubner, 1901) as the *Mulomedicina Chironis*.)

Our basic sources for the Roman practice of veterinary medicine come from the Byzantine era, and the *Corpus Hippiatricorum Graecorum* was collected in the ninth century under the direction of Constantine VII Porphyrogenitus, bringing together fragments from about 400 writers concerning the care of horses and their diseases as they had been assembled in the Hellenistic and Roman periods. The earliest authorities represented are Apsyrtus, the chief army veterinary surgeon to Constantine the Great (*vid.* E. Oder, 'Apsyrtus. Lebensbild des bedeutendsten altgriechischen Veterinars', *Veterinärhistorisches Jahrbuch*, II (1926), 121–36, and G. Björck, 'Apsyrtus Julius Africanus et l'hippiatrique grecque', in *Universitetets Årsskrift*, IV (Uppsala, 1944), and Hierocles (fl. *c.* 400) who wrote a treatise on the care of horses and leaves 107 fragments in the collection of Porphyrogenitus. Theomnestes (fl. *c.* 375) gives a few fragments from his lost treatise. The *Geoponica*, also composed under Constantine Porphyrogenitus, contained a few materials on the diseases of many domestic animals, from dogs, horses, sheep and cattle, to pigs and goats. We have no knowledge of works in the Hellenistic tradition earlier than Apsyrtus and Theomnestes. The basic bibliography for the Byzantine veterinary works is found in J. Hussey, ed., *Cambridge Medieval History*, IV, part II (Cambridge, 1967), 460, 462. Literature on Roman veterinary medicine is limited: *vid.* K. Hoppe, *PWK*, XVI A, 503, and J. Svennung, *Untersuchungen zu Palladius* (1935). The text of Pelagonius is edited by M. Ihm (Teubner, 1892).

Archaeology indicates something of veterinary medicine in the Roman legion. 'Horse physicians' may have been common, as

IGRR, I, 1252 (*Hippiatros* from Egypt), A. Schober, *Die römischen Grabsteine von Noricum* (Vienna, 1923), 47, No. 99 (*Pequarius legionis*), *CIL*, III, 10428 (Septimius Julianus: *miles pequarius* in the Legio II Adiutrix), and *CIL*, III, 13386 (Septimius Bauleus: *eques capsarius* for an undetermined legion near Aquincum) show. *Vid.* W. Haberling, 'Die Tierärzte im römischen Heere', *Zeitschrift für Veterinärkunde*, XXII (1910), 409–19, and K. György, *Die ärztliche Denkmäler von Aquincum* (Budapest, no date; rpt. (?) 1967; in Hungarian with German title and summary).

NOTES

ABBREVIATIONS

Africa   T. W. Africa, *Science and the State in Greece and Rome*
                        (New York, 1968)
AGM   *Sudhoffs Archiv für Geschichte der Medizin*
AJA   *American Journal of Archaeology*
AJP   *American Journal of Philology*
AMH   *Annals of Medical History*
Anat. Rec.   *Anatomical Record*
BCH   *Bulletin de correspondance Hellénique*
BCL   *Bohn's Classical Library*
Below   K.-H. Below, *Der Arzt im römischen Recht* (Munich,
                        1953)
BGU   *Berliner griechische Urkunden* (Ägyptische Urkunden
                        aus den königlichen Museen zu Berlin), 1895–?
BHM   *Bulletin of the History of Medicine*
BMJ   *British Medical Journal*
Brock   A. J. Brock, trans., *Galen: On the Natural Faculties*
                        (Loeb, 1916, rpt. 1952)
CAH   *Cambridge Ancient History*
CE   *Chronique d'Egypte*
CIG   *Corpus inscriptionum Graecarum*
CIL   *Corpus inscriptionum Latinarum*
CJ   *Classical Journal*
CP   *Classical Philology*
CQ   *Classical Quarterly*
CS   *Ciba Symposia*
Dodds, *Anxiety*   E. R. Dodds, *Pagan and Christian in an Age of Anxiety*
                        (Cambridge, 1965)
Drabkin, trans.,   I. E. Drabkin, trans., *Caelius Aurelianus On Acute
  or Drabkin, *Caelius*   Diseases and On Chronic Diseases* (Chicago, 1950)
  Aurelianus
Duckworth, *Later Books* W. L. H. Duckworth, trans. from the Arabic, *Galen
                        On Anatomical Procedures. The Later Books.* Ed. M. C.
                        Lyons and B. Towers (Cambridge, 1962)
Edelstein, *Asclepius* E. and L. Edelstein, *Asclepius* (Baltimore, 1945), 2 vols

Galen	Cited (unless otherwise stated) from C. G. Kühn *Galenus opera omnia* (rpt. Hildesheim, 1965), 20 vols in 22
GR	*Greece and Rome*
Haberling	W. Haberling, *Die altrömischen Militärärzte* (Berlin, 1910)
HC	W. W. Tarn, *Hellenistic Civilisation* (New York, 1963)
Herzog	R. Herzog, 'Urkunden zur Hochschulpolitik der römischen Kaiser', *Sitzungsberichte der preussischen Akademie der Wissenschaften, Phil.-Hist. Klasse*, XXXII (1935), 967–1019
Hopkins	K. Hopkins, 'Contraception in the Roman Empire', *Comparative Studies in Society and History*, VIII (1965), 124–51
HSCP	*Harvard Studies in Classical Philology*
IG	*Inscriptiones Graecae*
IGRR	Cagnat and Lafaye, *Inscriptiones Graecae ad res Romanas pertinentes*
ILS	Dessau, *Inscriptiones Latinae selectae*
Introduction	G. Sarton, *Introduction to the History of Science* (Washington, 1927), Vol. I
Jaeger	W. Jaeger, *Paideia* (Oxford, 1939), 3 vols
JDAI	*Jahrbuch des deutschen archäologischen Instituts*
JHB	*Johns Hopkins Hospital Bulletin*
JHI	*Journal of the History of Ideas*
JHM	*Journal of the History of Medicine and Allied Sciences*
JHS	*Journal of Hellenic Studies*
JRS	*Journal of Roman Studies*
Kudlien	F. Kudlien, *Die Sklaven in der griechischen Medizin der klassischen und hellenistischen Zeit* (Wiesbaden, 1968)
LCL	*Loeb Classical Library*
Marrou	H. I. Marrou, *A History of Education in Antiquity* (New York, 1964)
May, *Parts*	M. T. May, trans., *Galen On the Usefulness of the Parts of the Body* (Ithaca, New York, 1968), 2 vols
Michler	M. Michler, *Die alexandrinischen Chirurgen* (Wiesbaden, 1968)
Milne	J. S. Milne, *Surgical Instruments in Greek and Roman Times* (Oxford, 1907)
MLA	*Bulletin of the Medical Library Association*
NJ	*Neue Jahrbücher für das klassische Altertum*
OGIS	W. Dittenberger, *Orientis Graeci inscriptiones selectae* (Leipzig, 1903–1905)

PAAS	*Proceedings of the American Academy of Sciences*
PIC²	*Comptes rendus du deuxième congrès international d'histoire de la médecine* (Paris, 1921)
PIC³	*Proceedings of the Third International Congress of the History of Medicine* (London, 1922)
PIC⁶	*VIᵐᵉ congrès international d'histoire de la médecine* (Leiden and Amsterdam, 1927)
PRS	*Proceedings of the Royal Society of Medicine* (Section of the History of Medicine)
PWK	Pauly-Wissowa-Kroll, *Realencyclopädie der klassischen Altertumswissenschaft* (Stuttgart, 1895–)
QS	*Quellen und Studien zur Geschichte der Naturwissenschaften und der Medizin*
RC	R. B. Welles, *Royal Correspondence in the Hellenistic World* (New Haven, 1934)
Richmond	I. A. Richmond, 'Roman Britain and Roman Military Antiquities', *Proceedings of the British Academy* XLI (1955), 297–315
Rose	H. J. Rose, *A Handbook of Latin Literature* (New York, 1960)
Rufus	C. Daremberg and E. Ruelle, *Oeuvres de Rufus d'Ephèse* (Paris, 1879; rpt. Amsterdam, 1963)
Sarton, *Galen*	G. Sarton, *Galen of Pergamon* (Lawrence, Kansas, 1954)
SEG	*Supplementum Epigraphicum Graecum*
SEHHW	M. Rostovtzeff, *Social and Economic History of the Hellenistic World* (Oxford, 1941), 3 vols
SEHRE	M. Rostovtzeff, *Social and Economic History of the Roman Empire* (Oxford, 1957), 2 vols
SHA	*Scriptores historiae Augustae*
SIG³	W. Dittenberger, *Sylloge inscriptionum Graecarum.* 3rd edn (Leipzig, 1915–1924)
Singer, *Procedures*	C. Singer, trans., *Galen On Anatomical Procedures* (Oxford, 1956)
SMH	E. A. Underwood, ed., *Science, Medicine and History. Essays on the Evolution of Scientific Thought written in honour of Charles Singer* (Oxford, 1953), 2 vols
SPAW	*Sitzungsberichte der preussische Akademie der Wissenschaften, Phil.-Hist. Klasse*
Stahl	W. H. Stahl, *Roman Science* (Madison, 1962)
TAPA	*Transactions of the American Philological Association*
Temkin, *Soranus*	O. Temkin, trans., *Soranus' Gynecology* (Baltimore, 1956)
Vogt	J. Vogt, 'Wege zur Menschlichkeit in der antiken

Sklaverei', *Tübingen Rektoratsrede* (May 9, 1958),
19–38. Rptd in M. I. Finley, ed., *Slavery in Classical
Antiquity* (Cambridge, 1964), 33–52

Wilson   D. R. Wilson, 'Roman Britain in 1964: Sites Ex-
                plored', *JRS*, LV (1965), 199–220

WJ   *Würzburger Jahrbücher für die Altertumswissenschaft*

CHAPTER I

1 E. Gjerstad, *Legends and Facts of Early Roman History* (Lund, 1962), indicates
   the scepticism which accompanies archaeological comparison with legend-
   ary evidence. D. H. Trump, *Central and Southern Italy Before Rome* (London,
   1966), T. E. Peet, *The Stone and Bronze Ages in Italy* (Oxford, 1909), and
   A. M. Radmilli, *La Preistoria d'Italia alla luce delle ultime scoperte* (Florence,
   1963), show the painstaking efforts to elucidate early Italian history and
   culture. Early Rome and its connections with other major cultures in early
   Italy are shown in A. Alföldi, *Early Rome and the Latins* (Ann Arbor, 1965),
   and E. T. Salmon, *Samnium and the Samnites* (Cambridge, 1967). Still
   standard is J. Whatmough, *The Foundations of Roman Italy* (London, 1937).
2 Cicero, *Laws*, II, 7
3 Plutarch, *Numa*, 3. 6
4 Cicero, *On the Nature of the Gods*, III, 18
5 Cicero, *On Divination*, I, 9. 15
6 W. A. Jayne, *The Healing Gods of Ancient Civilizations* (rpt. New York,
   1962), 373–81
7 H. J. Rose, *Religion in Greece and Rome* (New York, 1960), 169
8 Livy, III, 7. 7–8
9 R. M. Ogilvie, *Commentary on Livy, Books I–V* (Oxford, 1965), 409
10 Tacitus, *Histories*, I, 63, also uses *stratae matres*. Apuleius, *Metamorphoses*, VI,
   2, employs *crinibus verrere* to show the meekest supplication
11 *Pacem* or *veniam exposcere* occurs also in Livy, I, 16. 3; III, 5. 14; IV, 30, 10;
   VII, 2. 2; XLIV, 44. 4, as it does in Catullus, 64. 203, Vergil, *Aeneid*, IV, 261,
   and Valerius Maximus, I, 1. 1. Ogilvie, 409
12 Ogilvie, 394–5
13 Livy, III, 8. 1
14 Pliny, XXIX, 5. 11
15 H. Gossen, 'Superstition in Roman Medicine', *CS*, I (May, 1939), 27–8.
   W. B. McDaniel, 'A Sempiternal Superstition', *CJ*, XLV (1950), 171–6,
   233–6. W. H. S. Jones, 'Ancient Roman Folk Medicine', *JHM*, XII (1957),
   459–72. Stahl, 106
16 W. H. R. Rivers, *Medicine, Magic and Religion* (London, 1924), 4.
17 H. Sigerist, *A History of Medicine* (Oxford, 1951), I, 114

M

18 X. F. M. G. Wolters, *Notes on Antique Folklore* (Amsterdam, 1935), 110
19 'head first'
20 'feet first'
21 Aulus Gellius, XVI, 16. 4
22 W. W. Fowler, *Roman Festivals* (London, 1899), 290–2
23 W. H. S. Jones, 'Roman Folk Medicine', *JHM*, XII (1957), 461
24 Cato, 83. This assertion has broad implications. Not only is the slave in the early Republic seen to be knowledgeable and able to perform the magico-medical rites as an integral part of the Roman household, but he is also a slave of a different nature than would be expected in the Greek world. C. Stace, 'The Slaves of Plautus', *GR*, s.s. XIV (1968), 64–77, argues from material in Plautus that such slaves, as existed on the Roman farm, show a stereotype, and that 'minor slaves must certainly be more like their Greek counterparts' [p. 76]
25 Cato, 132
26 Cato, 141
27 Cato, 134
28 Fustel de Coulanges, *The Ancient City* (New York, no date, trans. of W. Small [1873]), 89–90. Rose, *Religion*, 169–71
29 Horace, *Satires*, II, 3. 288
30 Pliny, XXIX, 8. 15–16
31 W. W. Buckland, *Textbook of Roman Law* (2nd edn, Cambridge, 1932), 585. F. de Zulueta, *The Institutes of Gaius* (Oxford, 1953), II, 209 [287 BC]
32 H. F. Jolowicz, *Historical Introduction to the Study of Roman Law* (Cambridge, 1952), 289
33 *Digest*, 9. 2. 7. 1. 8, 9 pr; 11 pr. F. Schulz, *Principles of Roman Law* (Oxford, 1956), 58–64. D. Daube, *Forms of Roman Legislation* (Oxford, 1956), 2
34 Pliny, XXIX, 8. 15
35 This would be a poultice made from one of the strongly scented plants of the genus *Ruta*, particularly *R. graveolens*
36 Pliny, XXIX, 9. 30–2
37 Pliny, XXIX, 9. 32
38 Suint is the natural grease of sheep wool, consisting of a mixture of fatty matter and potassium salts
39 Pliny, XXIX, 10–39
40 Cato, 156–8
41 Pliny, XXIX, 9. 30
42 Cato, 70. Trans. W. D. Hooper (*LCL*)
43 C. Bellini, 'A Farmer's Medical Prescription 2200 Years Ago', *CJ*, XLVIII (1952), 3–10. K. Barwick, 'Zu den Schriften des Cornelius Celsus und des alten Cato', *WJ*, III (1948), 117–32
44 The 'Hymn of the Arval Priests', *CIL*, I, 2nd edn, 2, and *CIL*, VI, 2104
45 Cato, 160
46 Cato, 127. 1–2. H. Wagenvoort, *Roman Dynamism* (Oxford, 1947)

47 R. Bloch, *The Origins of Rome* (London, 1963), 122–48, and *The Etruscans* (London, 1965), 142–60

48 The standard work on divination, though in some sections dated, is A. Bouché-Leclerq, *Histoire de la divination dans l'antiquité*, 4 vols (Paris, 1879–88). R. Bloch, *Les prodiges dans l'antiquité classique (Grèce, Étrurie et Rome)* in *Mythes et Religions* (Paris, 1962), gives a good summary of omens and their meaning. Cicero, *On Divination*, XXIII, tells the story of how Tages taught the Etruscans the art of divination. The problem of Etruscan origin is highly controversial. M. Pallottino, *The Etruscans* (Baltimore, 1955), believes these practices were a part of normal native development, running back to the Villanovans and before. Bloch, *Etruscans*, feels that the traditional account of the origins of the Etruscans in Asia Minor is reliable. H. H. Scullard, *The Etruscan Cities and Rome* (London, 1967), 17–19, does not believe either side has evidence strong enough for positive assertion. Proof of Phoenician involvement in early Italy is provided by the Pyrgi Inscriptions, described in J. Heurgon, 'The Inscriptions of Pyrgi', *JRS*, LVI (1966), 1–15, and Scullard, *Etruscan Cities*, 102–4

49 Pliny, II, 53–6 [138–46]. Seneca, *Quaestiones Naturales* [Budé], II, 32, 41, and 48. Cicero, *On Divination*, XXIII, and *On the Response of the Soothsayers*, II, 4, and III, 4–5, as well as many scattered references in Livy [particularly Bks. V and VII]

50 Scullard, *Etruscan Cities*, 68–9

51 M. Tabanelli, *Gli 'ex-voto' poliviscerali Etruschi e Romani* (Florence, 1962), plates 2, 6, 9, 16–29, and p. 86

52 G. Furlani, 'Mantica Hittita e Mantica Etrusca', *Studi Etruschi*, X (1936), 1–12, and 'L'epatoscopia babilones e l'epatoscopia etrusca', in *Atti del Primo Congresso Internaz. Etrusco* (Florence, 1929), 122–66

53 A. Bossier, 'Les Présages de Sargon et de Naram-Sin. Extraits des livres des haruspices', *Revue Sémitique*, X (1902), 275–80

54 G. Contenau, *La divination chez les Assyriens et les Babyloniens* (Paris, 1940), 242

55 M. Jastrow, 'The Liver as the Seat of the Soul', in *Studies in the History of Religion Presented to C. H. Toy* (New York, 1912), 143–68, and general remarks in his 'The Liver in Antiquity and the Beginnings of Anatomy' [an address delivered before the College of Physicians of Philadelphia, November 6, 1907], rptd in the University of Pennsylvania *Medical Bulletin* (1907)

56 Contenau, *Divination*, 257–68

57 Sigerist, *History*, I, 461

58 A. Ungnad, *Die Religion der Babylonier und Assyrier* (Jena, 1921), 312–20

59 A. Bossier, *Choix de textes relatifs à la divination assyro-babylonienne* (Geneva, 1905), I, 65 and 69ff

60 Sigerist, *History*, I, 462, quoting from Bossier, *Choix de textes*, I, 65–75. Sigerist, *History*, I, 472–7, provides a good bibliography for problems of divination in the ancient near east

61 M. Tabanelli, *La medicina nel mondo degli Etruschi* (Florence, 1963), 74–96 [with illustrations]. P. Deconfle, *La Notion d'ex-voto anatomique chez les Etrusco-Romains*, Collection Latomus Vol. LXXII (Brussels, 1964)

62 K. B. Maxwell-Hyslop, 'Urartian Bronzes in Etruscan Tombs', *Iraq*, XVIII (1956), 150ff

63 Tabanelli, *Medicina*, 84–5, 89

64 C. G. Leland, *Etruscan Magic and Occult Remedies* (rpt. New York, 1963), contends that Etruscan magical and medical practices are still in use in modern Tuscany, and that one can observe Etruscan themes in action

65 Ovid, *Fasti*, VI, 101–65

66 Cicero, *On the Nature of the Gods*, III, 63

67 Plautus, *Amphitryon*, V, 36–7, 39–42. Medical references in Plautus are collected in A. Spallaci, *La medicina in Plauto* (Milan, 1938)

68 E. Beneviste, 'La doctrine médicale des Indo-Européens', *Revue de l'Histoire des Religions*, CXXX (1945), 5–12. J. Filliozat, *The Classical Doctrine of Indian Medicine: Its Origins and Greek Parallels* (New Delhi, 1964)

69 Celsus, III, 23; IV, 7. 5, 13. 3; V, 28. 7B. Pliny, XXVIII, 2. 4

70 Celsus, IV, 9. 7

71 Celsus, III, 23

72 Scribonius Largus, XVII

73 Scribonius Largus, XIII

74 Serenus Sammonicus, *Liber Medicinalis* [ed. Pépin], L, 8–9 [930–1]

75 Serenus Sammonicus, XLIX [914–22]. Parallels for the remedy are in Pliny, XX, 155, XXIX, 61–3, and XXX, 99

76 Seneca, *Letters*, 95. 9–10, 15–16, 21

77 O. W. von Vacano, *The Etruscans in the Ancient World* (London, 1960), 137–49

78 Polybius, III, 22. *vid.* F. W. Walbank, *Historical Commentary on Polybius* (Oxford, 1957), I, 337–45, and Vol. II (Oxford, 1967), 635–6. The Punic-Etruscan Pyrgi Inscriptions seem to anchor the Polybian date of 509 BC for the first treaty. *Cf.* Note 48 above

79 von Vacano, 132. Pindar, *Pythian Odes*, I, 71–5. J. Boardman, *The Greeks Overseas* (Baltimore, 1964), 209–15

80 Macrobius, *Saturnalia*, I, 17. 14–16. Apollo could be the saviour-god at the same time as he sent the plague. T. Whittaker, *Macrobius* (Cambridge, 1923), 23

81 Livy, X, 47. Valerius Maximus, I, 8. 2. Ovid, *Metamorphoses*, XV, 622–744. Anonymous, *On Famous Men*, XXII, 1–3. The Greek Asclepius was known as Aesculapius in Rome, and sometimes the Italic goddess Salus was associated with the cult. Livy, XL, 37. J. Toutain, *Les cultes païens dans l'Empire Romain* (Paris, 1907), I, 330–8

82 Ovid, *Fasti*, I, 289–94. J. le Gall, 'Tiberina', *Revue Archéologique*, XLVII (1956), 34–44

83 Plutarch, *Numa*, is a clear indication

84 The dynamic influence of the cult was indeed long-lived. Suetonius, *Claudius*, 25. Augustine, *City of God*, III, 16. Arnobius, *Adverses Nationes*, VII, 44-8, and Claudian, *On the Consulship of Stilicho*, III, 171-3. The standard work on the cult of Asclepius in the Greek world is E. J. and L. Edelstein, *Asclepius* (Baltimore, 1945, 2 vols.). Epidaurus is considered in R. Herzog, *Die Wunderheilungen von Epidaurus* (Leipzig, 1931)

85 Their story will be considered in Chapter III below

86 Pliny, XXIX, 6. Hemina was an antiquarian who lived around 146 BC and wrote a history, or more correctly an anecdotal narrative, on the period down to his own day. His fragments are in H. Peter, *Historicorum Romanorum fragmenta* (Leipzig, 1883), 68-74. Cicero, *On the Orator*, II, 51-3, notes his brevity

87 Edelstein, *Asclepius*, I, 431-52, and II, 251-5

CHAPTER II

1 In this survey, Hippocratic medicine will not be considered, except as background for general discussion. The best account of the Hippocratic medical development (in English) is found in H. Sigerist, *A History of Medicine* (Oxford, 1961), II, 213-33. Of great importance are L. Edelstein, 'Hippocratic Prognosis', 'The Hippocratic Physician', 'The Role of Eryximachus in Plato's *Symposium*', 'Greek Medicine and Its Relation to Religion and Magic', and 'The Professional Ethics of the Greek Physician', in O. and C. Lilian Temkin, eds, *Ancient Medicine: Selected Papers of Ludwig Edelstein* (Baltimore, 1967)

2 Aristotle, *De Respiratione*, 480 b22

3 W. Jaeger, *Diokles von Karystos* (Berlin, 1938; rpt. 1963), 165

4 Jaeger, *Diokles*, 176. L. Edelstein in a review of Jaeger's *Diokles*, in *AJP*, LXI (1940), 483-9, denies Jaeger's new chronological position (*c.* 340-260 BC) for Diocles, but accepts the proposition that Diocles was at least contemporaneous with Aristotle, and that both had influence on one another. Aristotle exerted the greater influence. Edelstein acknowledges Jaeger's work as important, placing Diocles in a new position within philosophy so as to clarify Diocles' influence

5 L. Cohn-Haft, *The Public Physicians of Ancient Greece* (Northampton, Massachusetts, 1956), 4, 61-5. F. Kudlien, *Die Sklaven in der griechischen Medizin der klassischen und hellenistischen Zeit* (Wiesbaden, 1968), 35-8. *Cf.* C. A. Forbes, 'The Education and Training of Slaves in Antiquity', *TAPA*, LXXXVI (1955), 321-60, esp. 344

6 Kudlien, *Sklaven*, 37

7 Hyginus, *Fabulae*, 274, 10

8 M. Michler, *Die hellenistische Chirurgie*, Teil I: *Die Alexandrinischen Chirurgen* (Wiesbaden, 1968), 5-16

9 Marrou, 258

10 Athenaeus, VI, 268a; X, 424e

11 *Asclepius*, I. I. O. Deubner, *Das Asklepion von Pergamon* (Berlin, 1938), gives indication of the widespread influence such temple medicine had in late Hellenistic and Roman times at Pergamon. G. Sarton, *Galen of Pergamon* (Lawrence, Kansas, 1954), notes the influence the shrine had in the second century, and Aelius Aristides, *Sacred Tales*, gives a fascinating picture of the sort of hypochondria the shrine seemed to promote in Roman Asia Minor. [Aelius Aristides is considered at greater length in Chapter VII below]

12 V. Leonardos, 'Amphaireion skaphai', *Ephemeris Archaiologike* (1916), 118–21 [in Modern Greek], shows and analyses a votive bas-relief found in the Amphaireum, which indicates the usual combination of scientific and religious medicine in this period. The rational approach of the Hippocratic 'school' may be seen in passages from *On Diseases*, in particular II, 5 and 45. E. F. Cordell, 'Aretaeus the Cappadocian', *JHB*, XX (1909), 371–7, thinks that such passages point to Hippocratic auscultation of the heart

13 Cohn-Haft, *The Public Physicians of Ancient Greece*, makes it clear that one may not compare these 'public' physicians to the modern concept. Cohn-Haft argues that the individual doctor received an annually renewable income from a given city or Greek state, on the condition that he remain in the city. Doctors were 'migratory' as they had been earlier in Greek history. Private practice was carried on by the same individuals and they charged fees. The inscriptional evidence supports Cohn-Haft's point of view, although he appears to be needlessly harsh on the Greek practitioners. R. Pohl, *De Graecorum medicis publicis* (Berlin, 1905), is a convenient collection of most of the relevant inscriptions, although his conclusions are modified by Cohn-Haft's study

14 *SEHHW*, II, 1089

15 Thucydides, II, 52

16 *SIG³*, 943. *IG*, IX, 1. 516, and XII, 1. 1032

17 Inscriptions found on Cos indicate a wide scattering of Coan doctors in service in the Hellenistic world. R. Herzog, 'Vorläufiger Bericht über die archäologische Expedition auf der Insel Kos im Jahre 1902', *JDAI*, XVIII (1903), 1–12 [esp. 11], summarizes some of the inscriptions. *SIG³*, 528, adds further evidence to this point [dated *c*. 221–219 BC]. Related inscriptions from Gortyn and Delos appear in L. Laurenzi, 'L'Odeion di Coo', *Historia*, V (1931), 593–626 [esp. 620–2]. Further evidence is listed in *SEHHW*, III, 1598, and *HC*, 109–10, which gives proof from the Greek mainland. Greek medical 'schools' are surveyed in G. E. Gask, 'Early Medical Schools: Cyrene, Cos, and Cnidus', *AMH*, II (1940), 15–21. Cnidian medicine is considered to have heavy Egyptian backgrounds in J. B. de C. M. Saunders, *The Transitions from Ancient Egyptian to Greek Medicine* (Lawrence, Kansas, 1963)

18 Jardé, 'Inscriptions de Delphes', *BCH*, XXVI (1902), 246–86 [esp. 269–72 (218/217 BC)]. *SEHHW*, III, 1598

19 *SEHHW*, II, 1089. Polybius, V, 56–8. C. Gortemann, 'Médecine de cour dans l'Égypte du IIIᵉ siècle av. J. C.'. *CE*, XXXII (1957), 313–36. T. S. Brown, 'Apollophanes and Polybius, Book V', *Phoenix*, XV (1961), 187–95

20 *PWK*, V, col. 1155. *IG*, II, 946 [dated to 166/165 BC]. *OGIS*, 220 [dated to *c.* 270 BC]. Welles, *RC*, 64. The mention of an *archiatros* of Antiochus IX Cyzicenus occurs in *OGIS*, 256

21 Illustrative is the collection of medical tools found at Colophon, and dated to the Hellenistic era. R. Caton, 'Notes on a Group of Medical and Surgical Instruments found near Colophon', *JHS*, XXIV (1914), 114–18, with plates X–XIII. *Cf.* R. J. Forbes, 'New Data on Ancient Metallurgy', *Sibrium*, II (1955), 56–7, and E. H. Schulz, 'Zur Frage der Entwicklung des Stahles für ärztliche Instrumente', *AGM*, XXXIX (1955), 30–4

22 Theophrastus, *Historia plantarum*, IX, 16. 8, and 17

23 Teles, 18. Archaeological evidence for Hellenistic pharmaceuticals is common as suggested by E. Sjöquist, 'Morgantina: Hellenistic Medicine Bottles', *AJA*, LXIV (1960), 78–83

24 *OGIS*, 104

25 *SEHHW*, II, 1090

26 H. Opperman, 'Herophilus bei Kallimachos', *Hermes*, LVI (1925), 14–32. H. W. Miller, 'Medical Terminology in Tragedy'. *TAPA* (1944), 157–67. S. A. Wunderlich, 'Greek Art and Greek Medicine', *MLA*, XXXII (1944), 324–31, suggests that doctors and artists received similar training in anatomy. It is probable that some medical terminology was in widespread use among the educated in the Hellenistic world, as is argued by W. K. Hobart, *Medical Language in Luke* (Grand Rapids, Michigan [photostatic rpt. of 1882 edn] 1954). The contention is rejected by G. A. Lindeboom, 'Luke the Evangelist and the Ancient Greek Writers on Medicine', *Janus*, LII (1965), 144–8

27 *SEHHW*, II, 1091

28 *HC*, 187–8

29 *SEHHW*, I, 286; II, 1092–3

30 Herodotus, II, 84

31 K. Sudhoff, *Ärtzliches aus griechischen Papyrus-Urkunden* (Berlin, 1909), 252–79. C. Préaux, *L'Économie royale des Lagides* (Paris, 1938), 45, 132–40

32 Athenaeus, I, 3 a–b; V, 203e

33 E. G. Turner, 'L'érudition alexandrine et les papyrus', *CE*, XXXVII (1962), 135–52

34 Athenaeus, I, 22d. The early Roman imperial playwright, Antidotus, introduced on the stage a character like the modern professors (νῦν σοφιστεύουσιν) who reside at the Claudian Institute, 'whom it is disgraceful but to mention. This is what [Antidotus] says about the School of Parasites. . . .' (Athenaeus, VI, 240b–c.) Suetonius, *Claudius*, 42

35 O. Neugebauer in review of W. H. Stahl, *Roman Science* (Madison, 1962), in *AJP*, LXXXV (1964), 418–23 [esp. 420]. He adds [420], 'It is sad to see that

such are the results of penetrating studies of the Hellenistic world by generations of scholars.'

36 J. E. Sandys, *A History of Classical Scholarship* (rpt., New York, 1958), I,
110–12

37 Diodorus Siculus, III, 36. 3f

38 Galen, XVII, 1, 606. There were two libraries: the Brucheion, in the north-
eastern quarter close to the Museum, or in the western part (*cf.* Aristides
[Dindorf], II, 450), and the so-called 'daughter-library' in the south-western
quarter near to the Temple of Serapis. Sandys, *Classical Scholarship*, I, 107–9

39 Galen, XVII, 1, 607

40 *Greek Anthology*, VI, 270. Other epigrams attributed to Nicias are *Greek
Anthology*, VI, 122, 127; VII, 200; IX, 315, 564

41 A. S. F. Gow, *Theocritus* (Cambridge, 1952), I, xix, note 3, and II, 210 (XI, 7)

42 Gow, II, 208

43 Plutarch, *Spartan Sayings*, 218F (in period of Archidamus III, son of Agesi-
laus, king of Sparta, 361–338 BC). The question is posed to Periander, the
physician, 'Why do you ardently desire to be called a bad poet rather than a
good physician?'

44 Hippocrates: Apollonius of Citium wrote 18 books refuting Heracleides'
commentaries on Hippocrates [Erotian (ed. Klein), p. 32, 1]. Zenon, a
Herophilean (*c.* 200 BC), wrote two books in commentary on medical
histories in Hippocrates [Galen, XVII, 1, 618]. Cookery: Erasistratus wrote
a book on the *Art of Cookery* [Athenaeus, XII, 516d; VII, 324a]. Philistion of
Locris (fl. *c.* 380 BC) wrote on *Art of Cookery* [Athenaeus, XII, 516c]. Superstition: Andreas (physician to Ptolemy IV, killed at the Battle of Raphia,
217 BC [Polybius, V, 81. 6]), wrote *On Popular Superstitions* [Athenaeus, VII,
312e]. Perfumes: Apollonius Mys, a Herophilean, wrote a book *On Perfumes*
[Athenaeus, XV, 688e–689b; Pliny, XIII, 1. 2]. Wreaths: Philonides wrote a
treatise *On Perfumes and Wreaths* [Athenaeus, XV, 675a, 676c, 691f].
Dieuches taught Numenius of Heracleia who wrote a treatise *On Banquets*
[Athenaeus, I, 5b]. Drugs: Philistion of Locris wrote *On Remedies* [Caelius
Aurelianus, *Chronic Diseases*, V, 1. 23]. Andreas wrote *On Poisonous Animals*
[Athenaeus, VII, 312e]. Diet: Menodorus, an Erasistratean, wrote books on
pumpkins, squash, cucumbers, and melons [Athenaeus, II, 59a]. Philistion of
Locris wrote a book on when one should drink [Caelius Aurelianus,
Chronic Diseases, III, 8. 147]. Hicesius wrote *On Materials for Food* [Athe-
naeus, III, 118b; XV, 681c]. Medical practice: Erasistratus wrote a book *On
General Practice* [Athenaeus, XV, 665e–6a]

45 Diocles of Carystos (fl. 360 BC) wrote *On Health* [Athenaeus, II, 61c], *Art of
Cookery* [Athenaeus, XII, 516c], *On Deadly Drugs* [Athenaeus, XV, 681b],
along with works on fish [Athenaeus, III, 110b, 116e; VII, 301 c, 305b, 309c,
316c, 319b, 320c, 326a, 329f (cf. Aristotle, *Parts of Animals*, 542b 35)],
crustaceans [Athenaeus, III, 105b–c], nuts of many varieties [Athenaeus II,
57b, 59b], and the properties of water [Athenaeus, II, 46d] and wine

[Athenaeus, I, 32d]. Tryphon of Alexandria (frg. 117 [ed. Velsen]) quotes Diocles on the qualities of bread. *Vid.* W. Jaeger, *Diokles* [Aristotle's school has heavy influence on Diocles]. Diphilus of Siphnos (fl. under king Lysimachus [Athenaeus, II, 51a]) wrote much; among his works were *On Salt Fish*, *On Food for Sick and Well*, and other treatises on beets, cabbage, carrots, berries and fruits, and nuts [Athenaeus, III, 120e–f; VIII, 355a–7a; IX, 369d, f, 371, a, b, e; XIV, 650b; II, 50b, 51a, f]

46 F. Steckerl, *The Fragments of Praxagoras and His School* (Leiden, 1958), for convenient summary of his medical writings. Diphilus' fragments appear in Athenaeus, *Deipnosophists*, as listed in note 45 above, and is not quoted by Galen, as are Praxagoras and Diocles

47 L. Edelstein, *The Idea of Progress in Classical Antiquity* (Baltimore, 1967), 27–40, 70–80, 105, 140–60

48 Theopompus' *Phineus* (*apud* Athenaeus, XIV, 649b) has a mock physician give a fake—but convincing—prescription for constipation. Athenaeus, XV, 665e–6a, is essentially an essay on the pun in Greek of ἀποκοτταβίζειν, which can mean 'quickly consume the last of the wine' or 'vomit'. In the discussion of the Deipnosophistae that follows, Erasistratus is quoted on his method of purging (to gulp wine all in one swig allows a purge of the stomach: it is vomited up) and the practice supposedly harms the eyes and blocks the intestines. Then (666a) one of the other 'doctors at dinner' remarks, 'If it weren't for the physicians, there would be no men more stupid than the grammarians'

49 Athenaeus, XII, 552c

50 Diogenes Laertius, VII, 186 (Chrysippus)

51 Ruled in Alexandria, 146–117 BC

52 Plutarch, *How to Tell a Flatterer from a Friend*, 17 (60A). In one of these discussions, Ptolemy proposed a clever emendation of a line from the *Odyssey* (V, 72) [Athenaeus, II, 61c]

53 Neugebauer, in Review of Stahl, *AJP*, LXXXV (1964), 420

54 J. F. Dobson, 'Herophilus of Alexandria', *PRS*, XVIII (1924), 19–32 [19]

55 Galen, VIII, 724; XVIII, 2, 13–14

56 Galen, I, 109; III, 21; V, 879, 898; X, 28; XIV, 683; XV, 134

57 Galen, XIX, 64–5

58 Galen, XV, 136. Marinus is praised again in Galen, II, 280–3, and XVIII, 2, 926. Numesianus figures in Galen's comments on the tradition of Hippocrates. Numesianus wrote tracts on Hippocrates. Galen, XVI, 197, and XIX, 57. Marinus and Numesianus were philosopher-physicians in the second century, contemporary with Galen's training period. Galen, XIX, 25–30 [Marinus]

59 Africa, *Science*, 50

60 M. Wellmann, 'Über Träume', *AGM*, XVI (1924), 70–2. *PWK*, XV, cols 1104–10. Herophilus thought of drugs as the 'hands of the gods' [Galen, XII, 966]. Celsus notes Herophilus always used drugs in treating diseases

(Celsus, V, prooemium, 1.). *Cf.* Caelius Aurelianus, *Chronic Diseases*, II, 13.
186

61 See Appendix III

62 Galen, II, 895–6

63 Galen, XIX, 315. The terse account shows the great difference of opinion among authorities on the topic [Herophilus, Democritus, Plato, Strato, Erasistratus, Parmenides, and Epicurus]

64 Galen, III, 665

65 Galen, II, 570 [liver]; III, 665–7 [heart]; XIX, 315 [brain]; VIII, 212; III, 813; V, 206 [nerves]. Galen, VII, 605, and XIX, 318, obscures some of this classification, but elsewhere (Galen, VIII, 645) notes that 'Herophilus says the strength of the "vital power" causes a vigorous pulse'. Rufus of Ephesus (Daremberg-Ruelle), 162 and 220, tells of Herophilus' work on the comparison of the structures of arteries and veins

66 Rufus, 171, 154. Celsus, VII, 7. 13. For some reason, Rufus' correct description was discarded and the erroneous representation appears in Vesalius' *De Fabrica*. *Cf.* J. Scarborough, 'The Classical Background of the Vesalian Revolution', *Episteme*, II (1968), 200–18

67 (Pulse refs): Rufus, 220, 224. Galen, VIII, 911–13; 592, 786, 556, 871, 955; IX, 453 [Herophilus wrote a treatise *On Pulsation* on which Galen comments]

68 Galen admits his heavy debt to Herophilus in anatomy [Galen, V, 155; VIII, 212; IX, 463; XIII, 79]. Some errors creep into Galen's account from Herophilus [II, 890: uterus with horns]

69 The sketch below is taken from Pliny, XXIX, 3; Galen, IV, 707; XI, 191; and Caelius Aurelianus, *Chronic Diseases*, II, 13. Galen, II, 105, in describing Erasistratus' system of biological waste, reminds one of the Heraclitean theory of flux and change of one object into another

70 Galen, IV, 707

71 Galen, V, 602

72 Rufus, 164. Galen, V, 602–3. Erasistratus did comparative studies, noting the difference between the complexity of man's brain and those of lower animals. Galen, III, 673

73 D. Fleming, 'Galen on the Motions of the Blood in the Heart and the Lungs', *Isis*, XLVI (1955), 14–21. Galen, XI, 153; VIII, 311 [possible knowledge of pulmonary circulation]. Galen, V, 562 [heart as pump]

74 Galen, III, 492; IV, 706–8

75 Plato, *Timaeus*, 91

76 Galen, III, 537–9

77 Galen, XV, 306 [nerve]; XI, 147, 153 [vein]

78 Caelius Aurelianus, *Chronic Diseases*, III, 4. 65

79 Athenaeus, IV, 184c, quoting from Menecles of Barca and Andrion of Alexandria

80 M. Wellmann, 'Zur Geschichte der Medizin im Alterthume', *Hermes*, XXIII (1888), 556–66

81 Galen, XIII, 462; XII, 989; XVIII, 1, 735

82 Zenon: Galen, XVII, 1, 168. Mantias: Galen, XIII, 462. Serapion: Caelius
Aurelianus, *Chronic Diseases*, I, 4. 137–9. K. Deichgräber, *Die griechische
Empirikerschule* (rpt., Berlin, 1965), 258, 401. Serapion wrote a treatise
Against the Sects which 'obscura nimium atque pauca ordinavit, quorum
nihil est dignum enarrare'. Caelius Aurelianus, *Acute Diseases*, II, 6. 32.
Wellmann, 'Zur Geschichte', 559–60, remarks, '. . . the older medical literature was not disregarded by Serapion'. Philotimus: Caelius Aurelianus,
Acute Diseases, II, 16. 96: *Chronic Diseases*, I, 4. 140. Evenor: Pliny, XXI,
105, 180; XX, 73. 187, 191. Caelius Aurelianus, *Acute Diseases*, II, 16. 96.
Nileus: Caelius Aurelianus, *Acute Diseases*, II, 29. 153; *Chronic Diseases*, II,
1. 34. Molpis, Nymphodorus, Andreas, Protarchus: form common source
for Galen, XVIII, 1, 731, and Celsus, VIII, 20. 4, via Heracleides of Tarentum. Wellmann, 'Zur Geschichte', 560

83 Celsus, V, 18. 6. Galen, XIII, 220, 979

84 *PWK*, XV, cols 493–6 on Heracleides of Tarentum, and XIII, 1399, on
Glaucias of Tarentum. M. Michler, 'Das Problem der westgriechischen
Heilkunde', *AGM*, XLVI (1962), 137–52

85 M. Laignel-Lavastine, 'Influence de l'esprit libéral de Darius 1er dans les
relations médicales Indo-Helléniques avant Alexandre', *Actes VIIe Congrès
International d'Histoire des Sciences*, II (1950), 4–12. Appian, XI, 10. 59–61,
tells the famous story of Erasistratus and Seleucus

86 Filliozat, *Classical Doctrine of Indian Medicine*. W. W. Tarn, *The Greeks in
Bactria and India* (Cambridge, 1951), is not so sure of the Greek influence in
Indian medicine. He reflects that there is much disagreement among authorities [pp. 385–6]. M. Winternitz, *Geschichte der indischen Literatur* (1920), III,
554 [Tarn, note 4, p. 385], agrees with Filliozat, but A. B. Keith, *The
Sanscrit Drama* (1924), 513–14 [Tarn, note 1, p. 386], feels that no conclusion
on the problem is possible. For Indian medicine, see Sigerist, II, 121–96,
with bibliographical references. H. R. Zimmer, *Hindu Medicine* (Baltimore,
1948), is a standard reference. W. Kirfel, 'Ist die altindische Medizin
Arischen Ursprungs?', *AGM*, XXXIX (1955), 363–78 [yes, plus Dravidian
influence]. R. F. G. Muller, 'Kannten die altindischen Ärzte die Lunge?',
AGM XXXIX (1955), 134–44 [no, at least not until much later]

CHAPTER III

1 'Pythagoreanism' in the medicine of Cato is an example. Cato, 157

2 Pliny, XXVI, 7–8; XXIX, 6. Celsus, III, 14

3 Pliny, XXVI, 6. 11

4 Pliny, XXVI, 6. 11–17. 1

5 Galen, XX (index), 71–2, lists over three full columns of references. *Cf.* Rufus, 112, 184, 574, 578–9, and Soranus, *Gynecology* (Temkin), I, 9. 35; III, pr. 2–4; III, 3. 29

6 Galen, II, 40

7 Pliny, XXVI, 7. 12–13

8 Galen, II, 40–1

9 Galen, II, 39: τοῦτο γὰρ ἦν δηλαδὴ μέγα καὶ σεμνὸν ἀπιστήσαντα τοῖς φαινομένοις πιστεῦσαι τοῖς ἀδήλοις. Pliny, XXVI, 8. 15–16: Id solum possumus indignari, unum hominem e levissima gente sine opibus ullis orsum vectigalis sui causa repenta leges salutis humano generi dedisse, quas tamen postea abrogavere multi

10 Pliny, XXVI, 7–9. *Anonymus Londinensis* (Jones), XXIV, 30. Pliny believed that Democritus was the chief exponent of the 'magic art' as Hippocrates was of the 'medical art'. K. Freeman, *Companion to the Pre-Socratic Philosophers* (Oxford, 1946), 323

11 Caelius Aurelianus, *Chronic Diseases*, III, 8, 149–51. Pliny, XXVI, 8. 17

12 Pliny, XXIX, 6. Cicero, *On the Orator*, I, 62. Celsus, III, 14. 2; 18. 5, 14–15. R. M. Green, *Asclepiades: His Life and Writings* (New Haven, 1955), 1–11. This is an English translation of Cocchi, *Life of Asclepiades* (Florence, 1762), and of Gumpert, *Fragments of Asclepiades* (Weimar, 1794), which I could not obtain. H. von Vilas, *Asklepiades von Bithynien* (Leipzig, 1903), 11–15

13 Dropsy: the modern medical definition is an excessive accumulation of clear watery fluid in any of the tissues or cavities of the body. Borrowing: Celsus, III, 14; *Prooemium*, 11. Caelius Aurelianus, *Acute Diseases*, I, 14

14 Caelius Aurelianus, *Chronic Diseases*, V, 2. 51; *Acute Diseases*, III, 1. 5

15 Caelius Aurelianus, *Chronic Diseases*, III, 8. 149. Drabkin, trans., 809

16 Caelius Aurelianus, *Acute Diseases*, I, 14. 109–15. Drabkin, trans., 69–73

17 Celsus, *Prooemium*, 11

18 Celsus, *Prooemium*, 11. 'Et per hos quidem maxime viros salutaris ista nobis professio increvit'

19 Hippocrates, *Airs, Waters, Places*, XIV, 1–3: καὶ ὁκόσα μὲν ὀλίγον διαφέρει τῶν ἐθνέων παραλείψω, ὁκόσα δὲ μεγάλα ἢ φύσει ἢ νόμῳ, ἐρέω περὶ αὐτῶν ὡς ἔχει. Barbarian inferiority to the Greek is passed over. Strabo, I, 66. F. H. Heinimann, *Nomos und Physis* (Basel, 1945), 13–17

20 M. Hadas, 'From Nationalism to Cosmopolitanism', *JHI*, IV (1943), 105–11. M. Hadas, *Hellenistic Culture* (Oxford, 1959), 15–16: 'The arguments for human equality on the basis of a common *physis* received much wider dissemination through the Cynics and their street-corner preachers. . . . The Cynics were concerned for the happiness of the individual . . . the Stoics . . . thought primarily in terms of the community. . . . Relationships of blood or race or country are meaningless, political and social stratifications are rejected'

21 Jaeger, *Diokles*, 186–223. Celsus, *Prooemium*, 8 and 20

22 Celsus, VII, prooemium

23 As the Hellenistic patterns became accepted, even the 'theory' of medicine became a sort of question-and-answer session. Marrou, *History of Education*, 265, with reference to Geneva Papyrus 111

24 Rufus, 296. Galen, XVIII, 2, 631; XVII, 1, 826, 793 [Zeuxis]; Galen, III, 787 [Hicesius], and Strabo, XII, 8. 20

25 Again, it should be emphasized, these 'schools' were merely results of a generally informal influence of one medical teacher on his colleagues and students

26 Singer, *Procedures*, xvi–xvii

27 Galen, XIX, 228 [Pyrrho]. Diogenes Laertius, *Pyrrho*, IX, 106 [association of Pyrrhonic thought and Zeuxis]. L. Edelstein, 'Empirie und Skepsis in der Lehre der griechischen Empirikerschule', *QS*, III (1933), 253–78, and 'The Distinctive Hellenism of Greek Medicine', *BHM*, XL (1966), 197–225

28 R. Fuchs, 'Aus Themisons Werke über die akuten und chronischen Krankheiten', *Rheinisches Museum*, LVIII (1903), 67–114. Galen, IX, 476; X, 35; XIII, 40, 158, 1009; XIV, 648

29 Thessalus: T. Meyer-Steineg, 'Thessalos von Tralles', *AGM*, IV (1910), 89–108. Connection is drawn between Thessalus and Silius Italicus and his *Punica* by M. Neuburger, 'Medizinisches aus dem Epos des C. Silius Italicus "Punica"', *Eesti Arst*, IX (1924), 215–20. Along with Hellenistic-methodistic influence from Thessalus, the complex intellectual environment around Silius Italicus is seen by further references to Hellenistic borrowings. Tacitus, *Histories*, III, 65. Martial, VII, 63; VIII, 66; IX, 86; XI, 48, 50. He had some contact with the Stoic Epictetus. A. Bonhöffer, *Epiktet und die Stoa* (Giessen, 1890). Galen, X, 7, 8. Soranus: The best summary of Soranus, and those who preceded and followed him, is found in O. Temkin's introduction to his translation of Soranus' *Gynecology* (Baltimore, 1956). Caelius Aurelianus: Drabkin, *Caelius Aurelianus*, xi–xvii, reviews the Methodism of Caelius Aurelianus and his relationship to Soranus

30 M. Wellmann, *Die Pneumatische Schule bis auf Archigenes* (Berlin, 1895). Vol. XIV of *Philologische Untersuchungen*

31 Galen, I, 457; VII, 174; VIII, 748; X, 839; XII, 839. Wellmann, *Die Pneumatische Schule*. The Pneumatics may have had their inspiration from the medical centre at Pergamon. Oribasius, III, 688. 17. Caelius Aurelianus, *Chronic Diseases*, II, 7; *Acute Diseases*, II, 38. S. Sepp, *Pyrrhoneische Studien* (Freising, 1893), 120–2

32 Galen, I, 64–223, is devoted to two studies of the medical sects and their faults and virtues. Here Galen's dislike for the Methodists is seen at its harshest. As Sarton, *Galen*, 37, has aptly pointed out, Galen was able to 'see the weak points of other people's procedure, but his scientific education was too rudimentary to teach a general method . . . there was hardly a general method of science before the seventeenth century, and two more centuries would be needed to clarify and simplify it.' Galen's own Eclectic leanings are well seen in XIX, 13, where a Roman colleague of Galen, one Martialis, is

asked, 'To what sect does Galen belong?' and was answered: 'He belongs to none and calls slaves those who accept as final the teachings of Hippocrates or Praxagoras or anybody else.' (Sarton, trans., *Galen*, 37.) Thus Eclecticism offered no new approaches to the old questions; it merely rejected some of the old answers

33 Galen, VII, 295. Antyllus, who quotes Archigenes, and is quoted by Galen, shows the general development. Galen, II, 571. Aetius, VII, 46. J. Hirschberg, 'Die Star-Operation nach Antyllos', *Zentralblatt für praktische Augenheilkunde*, XXX (1906), 97–100, and R. L. Grant, 'Antyllus and his Medical Works', *BHM*, XXXIV (1960), 154–74

34 Aretaeus of Cappadocia (C. G. Kühn, ed., *Medicorum Graecorum Opera*, vol. XXIV [Leipzig, 1828]), 185, 209, 295. F. Kudlien, *Untersuchungen zu Aretaios von Kappadokien* (Wiesbaden, 1964), 11, 14–15, 24–6. The close relations with philosophical thought are shown in F. Kudlien, 'Poseidonios und die Ärzteschule der Pneumatiker', *Hermes*, XC (1962), 419–29

35 Galen, VIII, 203; X, 929. Oribasius, IV, 529

36 Miriam F. Drabkin and I. E. Drabkin, *Caelius Aurelianus. Gynaecia. Fragments of a Latin Version of Soranus' Gynaecia From a Thirteenth Century Manuscript* (Baltimore, 1951 [Supplements to *BHM* No. 13]). Caelius Aurelianus was a literal copyist of Soranus, omitting large sections, particularly the doxographical and historical material. Other sources behind Caelius Aurelianus are examined in G. Bendz, *Studien zu Caelius Aurelianus und Cassius Felix* (Lund, 1964)

37 M. Wellmann, 'Zu Herodots Schrift περὶ τῶν ὀξέων καὶ χρονίων νοσημάτων', *Hermes*, XLVIII (1913), 141. Wellmann has collected the fragments in 'Herodots Werk περὶ τῶν ὀξέων καὶ χρονίων νοσημάτων', *Hermes*, XL (1905), 580–604. Galen, XIV, 675–6, notes his originality in approaching medical problems. He was remembered for his use of physical agents where none had been used before

38 Oribasius, IV, 51. 564. The text used is from Wellmann, 'Herodots Werk', *Hermes*, XL (1905), 589–90. Cupping-glass; this is the *curcurbita*, or a glass or metal cup which was heated and applied to induce slow bleeding. [Her. σίκυα]

39 Aulus Gellius, *Attic Nights*, XVIII, 10: 'I, therefore, have used what time I could spare in reading certain medical handbooks which I thought appropriate to instruct me, and now, in addition to all sorts of other related things, I know the relationship between the arteries and veins. . . .'

40 Temkin, *Soranus*, xxxvii, *CIL*, II, 497, shows that women were highly valued in problems of this kind [*medica optima* from Emerita in Spain]

41 Temkin, *Soranus*, 129

42 *Ibid.*, 45–6

43 *Ibid.*, 5

44 Rufus of Ephesus, *On Interrogation of the Patient*, as trans. by A. J. Brock, *Greek Medicine* (London, 1929), 113. His text is Daremberg.

45 *Ibid.*, 124

46 Rufus, 297

47 Rufus, 291. Galen, II, 131

48 H. Flashar, *Melancholie und Melancholiker in den medizinischen Theorien der Antike* (Berlin, 1966), 73–83 [Celsus, Aretaeus, and Soranus], 84–104 [Rufus], and 105–17 [Galen]. *Cf.* R. F. Timken-Zinkann, 'Black Bile. A Review of recent Attempts to Trace the Origin of the Teachings on Melancholia to Medical Observations', *Medical History*, XII (1968), 288–92

49 Galen, II, 34

50 Galen, II, 35: οὕτως οὐ μόνον οὐδὲν ὑγιὲς ἴσασιν οἱ ταῖς αἱρέσεσι δουλεύοντες, ἀλλ᾽ οὐδὲ μαθεῖν ὑπομένουσι. 'Sects' does not quite capture the sense of the Greek, as it overdefines it. Something akin to 'clubs of men with similar opinions' would be closer. *Cf.* Singer, *Procedures*, xv

51 Singer, trans., *Procedures*, xxiii, with a list of passages in the treatise which might indicate a close acquaintance with human anatomy. In Galen, III, 423 (*De usu partium*, VI, 4), occurs a statement which apparently shows that Galen had dissected humans, but the context leaves doubt as to whether the line means 'explaining construction for men' or 'dissecting men'. It is certain that Galen's knowledge of bones was based on human material. *Vid.* Galen, II, 732–78 (*De ossibus ad tirones*), and Singer's translation in *PRS*, XLV (1952), 25–34

52 Singer, *Procedures*, xxiv

53 C. Singer, ed. and trans., *Vesalius On the Human Brain* (Oxford, 1952), xviii–xx, summarizes Galen's 'physiology'

54 Singer, trans., *Procedures*, 31

55 Singer, *Procedures*, 241

56 Freeman, *Companion to the Pre-Socratic Philosophers*, 289–326 (298, 308, 323–4, for medical references to Democritus) and *Ancilla to the Presocratic Philosophers* (Oxford, 1962), 91–120 [frgs. of Democritus]. Other names in this philosophic-medical tradition were Bolus of Mende (pp. 337–8, Freeman, *Companion*), Gorgias of Leontini (*ibid.*, 353–67), and Antiphon the Sophist (*ibid.*, 391–404, esp. 403–4)

57 Singer, trans., *Procedures*, 31–2

58 *Ibid.*, 34–6

59 Galen, VI, 29. I have taken some liberties with the Galenic prolixity, by expressing in relatively terse English the convoluted thoughts of the Greek. I have attempted to retain the 'wordy' tone

60 Galen, II, 27–34

61 Galen's writing appears to be a landmark in the debate between philosophical truth based on human reason, and the Hebrew and Christian concept of religious revelation from a supernatural agency. The debate goes on in our day with as little settlement between the 'mystics' and the 'intellectuals'. R. Walzer in *The Cambridge History of Later Greek and Medieval Philosophy*, ed. A. H. Armstrong (Cambridge, 1967), 646, 650, and his

fascinating *Galen On Jews and Christians* (Oxford, 1949). The tone of the age swung against Greek philosophy, but the debate continued throughout the middle ages. Stoicism had changed greatly since the days of Zeno, and we find prayers for the health of the soul coupled with bodily health (Seneca, *Letters*, X, 4, and Juvenal, X, 356), and Seneca bases his concept of happiness upon a continually healthy state of the mind (Seneca, *Dialogi*, VII, 3. 3). Chrysippus devoted great effort in comparing diseases of the soul to the body (Cicero, *Tusculan Disputations*, IV, 10. 23–4). *Cf.* J. S. Kieffer, trans., *Galen's Institutio Logica* (Baltimore, 1964), 9–12, and N. Rescher, *Galen and the Syllogism* (Pittsburgh, 1966), 8 and 65

62 Galen, II, 107, 117 (καὶ τούτῳ τῷ λόγῳ πάνθ' ὁμολογεῖ τὰ φαινόμενα), 118, 134–5

63 We must, however, not refer to the Byzantine period in the history of medicine as 'stagnant', simply because Byzantine history appears to reflect further consolidation of the classical ideal. *Vid.* O. Temkin, 'Byzantine Medicine, Tradition and Empiricism', *Dumbarton Oaks Papers*, XVI (1962), 95–115, D. J. Geanakoplos, *Byzantine East and Latin West* (New York, 1966), 29–31, L. Thorndike, 'Translations of Works of Galen from the Greek by Niccolo da Reggio (*c.* 1308–45)', *Byzantina-Metabyzantina*, I (1946), 213–35, and S. Eyice, 'The Practice of Medicine, Physicians, Institutions of Health in Byzantium during the Byzantine Period' (in Turkish with résumé in English), *İstanbul Üniv. Tip. Fak. mecmnasc*, XXI (1958), 657–91

64 Walzer, *Galen On Jews and Christians*, 1

CHAPTER IV

1 A. J. Toynbee, *Hannibal's Legacy* (Oxford, 1965), II, 384–5. Livy, XXIX, 14, tells the colourful story of the acceptance of Magna Mater into Rome. Toynbee, 386, calls Rome full of 'emotionally hungry masses'. The title of his chapter [XII, 374–415], 'Religious Response to Spiritual Ordeals', gives some idea of the tone. For a more balanced view, see H. Graillot, *Le culte de Cybèle Mère des Dieux, à Rome et dans l'Empire Romain* (Paris, 1912), 29–34. Graillot [23] notes that Magna Mater presented problems for Roman authorities as she had for civic leaders in Athens and Syracuse

2 Stahl, 65–83

3 J. Ilberg, 'A. Cornelius Celsus und die Medizin in Rom', *NJ*, XIX (1907), 376–412 [388]

4 W. H. S. Jones, 'Ancient Documents and Contemporary Life, with Special Reference to the Hippocratic *Corpus*, Celsus, and Pliny', *SMH*, I, 100–10 [105–6]

5 A casual glance at the *Tusculan Disputations* or *On Divination* shows many instances of adaptive originality

6 B. Meinecke, 'Aulus Cornelius Celsus: Plagiarist or Artifex Medicinae?', *BHM*, X (1941), 288–98. One instance of Celsus' synthetic skill is examined in K. Heinemann, 'Aus der Frühgeschichte der Lehre von den Drüsen im menschlichen Körper', *Janus*, XLV (1941), 137–65, 219–39 [Celsus' classification of glands]

7 A. D. Winspear, *Lucretius and Scientific Thought* (Montreal, 1963), 80–116. P. Ménière, *Etudes médicales sur les poètes latins* (Paris, 1858), 96–115

8 A. Castiglioni, 'Aulus Cornelius Celsus as a Historian of Medicine', *BHM*, VIII (1940), 859–73 [859]

9 T. J. Haarhof, *The Stranger at the Gate* (Oxford, 1948), 209–10, and A. N. Sherwin-White, *Racial Prejudice in Imperial Rome* (Cambridge, 1967), 71–7, use Juvenal to show a kind of cultural rivalry in Rome for patronage between Greeks and Romans

10 Pliny, XXIX, 7. 14

11 Plutarch, *Cato Major*, 3

12 *Ibid.*, 2–3, 23

13 Toynbee, *Legacy*, II, 106

14 E. V. Marmorale, *Cato Major* (Bari, 1949), 151

15 Plutarch, *Cato Major*, 12

16 Marmorale, 56–60

17 L. Alfonsi, 'Catone il Censore e l'umanismo romano', *La Parola del Passato*, IX (1954), 161–76 [168], and F. Della Corte, *Catone Censore* (Turin, 1949), 150–2, note this problem

18 Plutarch, *Cato Major*, 20. 8. Marcus married Lucius Aemilius Paullus' daughter, Tertia, and thus became the brother-in-law of Scipio Aemilianus. Della Corte, 60–80. A. E. Astin, *Scipio Aemilianus* (Oxford, 1967), 36

19 Toynbee, *Legacy*, II, 427, bases his assumption on De Sanctis, *Storia dei Romani*, IV, pt. II, t. i, 60

20 Nepos, *Cato*, III, 1: 'In omnibus rebus singulari fuit industria: nam et agricola sollers et peritus, iuris consultis et probabilis orator et cupidissimus litterarum fuit.' P. Reuther, *De Catonis de agri cultura libri vestigiis apud Graecos* (Leipzig, 1903)

21 Cato, *On Agriculture*, 4. 5. *Cf.* Livy, XXXII, 26, and Diodorus Siculus, XI, 25 [Agrigentum and Syracuse], XXII, 81 [Agrigentum], and XIII, 83 [Acragas]

22 184 BC. Livy, XXXIX, 44

23 Della Corte, 93–7

24 Suetonius, *Claudius*, 42. 1: 'Uterque sermo noster'

25 Toynbee, *Legacy*, II, ch. 13 (416–34)

26 Cato, 70–3, 101–4

27 Plutarch, *Cato Major*, 20. T. C. Allbutt, 'Greek Medicine in Rome: The Fitzpatrick Lectures', *BMJ* (1909), pt II, 1149–55, 1515–22, 1598–1606 [1453] has some cogent remarks: '. . . historians have done Cato some injustice . . . we . . . have derived our impressions of Cato from the babbling

N

of Pliny, who had the vanity and garrulity of Boswell without his reverential sincerity. . . . Cato was for his time a learned man . . . before Celsus and Varro, he was an encyclopedist—a "summist" whose chapters not only on military matters and agriculture but also on law and history, were extant and respected in Cicero's generation'

28 Pliny, XXV, 2, and XXIX, 6

29 Cato, 6–9, 157. 157 begins: 'De brassica Pythagorea, quid in ea boni, sit salubritatisque.' W. H. Roscher, *Die Hebdomadenlehren der griechischen Philosophen und Ärzte* (Leipzig, 1906), 41–6. Reuther, 33–40. The study of Pythagoreanism was the activity of Nigidius Figulus, a close friend of Cicero, who wrote in close alliance with biological and medical study. Aulus Gellius, IV, 9. 1 and 16, speaks of him as one of the great scholars next to Varro. The fragments of Figulus are collected in A. Swoboda, *P. Nigidii Figuli operum reliquiae* (Vienna, 1889; rpt. Amsterdam, 1964)

30 Varro, *On Agriculture*, I, 2. 28; I, 7. 1; I, 18. 1 [on slaves; differs from Cato]; I, 58; II, 4. 11

31 Roman custom: Varro, I, 2. 3. Vergil, *Georgics*, I, 233. Both use the division of the earth into five zones, as Eratosthenes taught. Hellenistic models: Varro, I, 18. 3; 19. 1 and 3. Connection with Mago's work is seen in Varro, I, 17. 3; II, 5. 18; and III, 2. 13. Varro, I, 39. 3, and Virgil, *Georgics*, II, 10–36, use Theophrastus, *Historia plantarum*, II, 1. Varro, II, 10. 8, resembles Plutarch, *Cato Major*, 20

32 Varro, I, 4. 1–5; II, 10. 10; II, 1. 21–3; II, 3. 8. Varro, I, 4. 4: 'Nec haec non deminuitur scientia. Ita enim salubritas, quae dicitur e caelo ac terra, non est in nostra potestate, sed in naturae, ut tamen multum sit in nobis, quo graviora quae sunt ea diligentia leviora facere possumus.' *Diligens* is used by Pliny, XIII, 7. 31, to describe 'the most learned investigators' of nature (*diligentissimi naturae*), and in the medical context in XXXII, 13. 26 (*diligentissimus medicinae*)

33 Galen, XIX, 8–11, and IX, 789–90

34 Pliny, XXIX, 5. 11: 'Mutatur ars cottidie totiens interpolis, et ingeniorum Graeciae flatu inpellimur . . .'

35 Galen, XVIII, 2, 257–8

36 Stahl, 134–233, Martianus Capella is the major example. Medical summaries of Pliny became common, but lists of drugs of all sorts were more common. Stahl examines only the west

37 P. Thielscher, 'Vitruv und die Lehre von der Ausbreitung des Schalles', *Das Altertum*, IV (1958), 222–8

38 Vitruvius, I, 1. 10; I, 4. 6; VI, 2. 3

39 Vitruvius, VIII, 3. 19. Trans. M. H. Morgan, *Vitruvius: The Ten Books On Architecture* (Dover rpt., 1960)

40 Vitruvius, VIII, 3. 17. Trans. Morgan

41 *Contra* Stahl, 92–6. Thielscher examines Vitruvius' competence and adaptive ability. Aristoxenus was Vitruvius' starting point for his ideas of acoustics.

W. Sackur, *Vitruv und die Poliorketiker* (Berlin, 1925), 4–10, speaks of Vitruvius as a 'universal man'. Thielscher notes that Plutarch, *Placita philosophorum*, IV, 19, writes of these theories of sound with less insight

42 A. Söllner, *Die hygienischen Anschauungen des römischen Architekten Vitruvius* (Jena, 1913), points this up well with references from Vitruvius. M. H. Morgan, 'On the Language of Vitruvius', *PAAS*, XLI (1906), 467–502 and 'The Preface of Vitruvius', *PAAS*, XLIV (1909), 149–75, bring emphasis upon the many sources Vitruvius may have consulted. E. Schramm, 'Erläuterung der Geschützbeschreibung bei Vitruvius', *SPAW*, X (1917), 718–34, notes Vitruvius' knowledge of warcraft

43 L. Edelstein, 'On Medical Education in Greece and Rome', *BHM*, XV (1944), 333–51 [343]. H. I. Marrou, *A History of Education in Antiquity* (New York, 1964), 165, 177, 263–5

44 W. G. Spencer in his translation of Celsus (*LCL*), I, xi–xii, lists some of the passages he considers indicating Celsus as an 'experienced medical practitioner'. His arguments are summarized in 'Celsus' De Medicina—A Learned and Experienced Practitioner upon what the Art of Medicine Could Then Accomplish', *PRS*, XIX (1926), 129–39. M. Wellmann represents the other extreme in his *A. Cornelius Celsus. Eine Quellenuntersuchung* (Berlin, 1913) as he argues that Celsus merely copied from a certain Cassius [E. Kind denies the hypothesis in a review of Wellmann in *Berliner Philologische Wochenschrift*, XXXIV (1914), 319–94]. Wellmann later changed his mind as seen in his 'A. Cornelius Celsus', *AGM*, XVI (1925), 209–13. The literature on Celsus is enormous and the fashion of late has been to emphasize the 'copyist' qualities of Celsus, but balanced views are presented in B. Meinecke, 'Aulus Cornelius Celsus—Plagiarist or Artifex Medicinae?', *BHM*, X (1941), 228–98, and O. Temkin, 'Celsus' "On Medicine" and the Ancient Medical Sects', *BHM*, III (1935), 249–64. J. Ilberg, 'A. Cornelius Celsus und die Medizin in Rome', *NJ*, XIX (1907), 377–412, surveys the complexities in the era of Celsus. The scholarly literature has many examples of Celsus the 'encyclopaedist'. M. Schanz, 'Über die Schriften des Cornelius Celsus', *Rheinisches Museum*, XXXVI (1881), 362–78; W. Krenkel, 'Celsus', *Das Altertum* IV (1958), 111–22; J. Finlayson, 'Celsus', *Glasgow Medical Journal*, XXXVIII (1892), 321–48; A. Dyroff, 'Der philosophische Teil der Enzyklopädie des Cornelius Celsus', *Rheinisches Museum*, LXXXIV (1939), 7–18; and K. Barwick, 'Die Enzyklopädie des Cornelius Celsus', *Philologus*, CIV (1960), 236–49, are examples. For the whole of Roman encyclopedism, F. Della Corte, *Enciclopedisti Latini* (Genoa, 1946), is good

45 Columella, *On Agriculture*, I, 8. 4; II, 2. 24–5; II, 9. 11; II, 11. 6; III, 1. 8; III, 2. 24–7 and 31; III, 17. 4: '. . . Iulius Atticus et Cornelius Celsus, aetatis nostrae celeberrimi auctores . . .'; IV, 1. 1; IV, 8. 1; IV, 28. 2; IV, 5. 5 [on treatment for plague in cattle]; VI, 14. 6 [on treatment for swollen necks in oxen]; VII, 2. 2; VII, 3. 11; VII, 5. 15 [on treatment of lung diseases in sheep]; VIII, 13. 2–3; IX, 6. 2–4; IX, 7. 2; IX, 11. 5; IX, 14. 6; IX, 14.

18–19 [the sections in Book IX are concerned with beekeeping]

46 Columella, II, 2. 15: '. . . cum alios tum etiam Cornelium Celsum, non solum agricolationis sed universae naturae prudentum virum. . .'. Gargilius Martialis, IV, 1, says of Celsus: 'Italicae disciplinae peritissimum'

47 Quintilian, XII, 11. 24: 'Cum etiam Cornelius Celsus, mediocri vir ingenio, non solum de his omnibus conscripserit artibus, sed amplius rei militaris et rusticae et medicinae praecepta reliquerit, dignus vel ipso proposito, ut *eum scisse omnia illa credamus.*' 'Mediocri' probably should be rendered 'not ordinary' rather than 'average', given the context of the passage. Quintilian makes use of Celsus' lost books on rhetoric [II, 15. 22 and 32; III, 1. 21]. Celsus had high standards in his discussion of oratory [III, 5. 3], and Quintilian recognizes Celsus' high level of intellect [III, 6. 38]. Quintilian's respect for Celsus is further illustrated in VII, 2. 19; VIII, 3. 35 [Celsus thinks orators ought not to coin new words]; VIII, 3. 47 [Celsus' knowledge of Greek noted, as well as a certain skill in double *entendre*]; IX, 1. 18 [Celsus' careful analysis of the *color* of a speech]; X, 1. 124 [praise for the philosophical works of Celsus]

48 Pliny cites Celsus twenty-four times; in Book I, Pliny lists his sources for each of the following books, and Celsus appears in the lists for Books VII–VIII, X–XI, XIV–XV, XVII–XXI (and by implication XXII), XXIII–XXIX, and XXXI. An example is Pliny, XX, 14. 29: 'Celsus et podagris quae sine tumore sint radicem eius in vino decoctam inponi iubet' [Celsus, IV, 31. 4]. Important in this reference is Pliny's use of *iubeo*, which implies authority. Pliny later says that 'the subject of medicine' has not been treated before in Latin [XXIX, 1. 1]. Pliny's concept of what Celsus had done is clear: Celsus operated as one of the traditional heads of the Roman household. Pliny distinguishes between the learned medical writers and the scholarly *medicus* that Celsus typified. Pliny's 'medical writers' are Greek (*vid.* source listings, Book I). Celsus clarifies his concept of the *medicus* in the Roman sense [*Prooemium*, 1–2]: 'Haec nusquam quidem non est siquidem etiam inperitissimae gentes herbas aliaque promta in auxilium vulnerum morborumque noverunt.' III, 6. 6: 'Ob quam causam periti medici est non potinus ut venit adprehendere manu brachium, sed primum disidere hilari vultu percontarique, quemamodum se habeat, et si quis eius metus est, eum probabili sermone lenire, tum deinde eius corpori manum admovere.' Celsus notes the tradition he stands in [I, 3. 22–3]; in III, 18, 4–5; V, 27. 3; VI, 6. 39; VII, prooemium, 1–2; VII, 2–4; and VIII, 4. 10–11, Celsus makes clear he adopts what is best from the 'ancients', whether Greek or Roman. The Roman *medicus* will have a *valetudinarium* ['recovery area for the ill'] which would be a part of the farm or aristocratic home [*Prooemium*, 65]. Veterinary medicine forms a section of the Roman *medicus-pater familas* [*Prooemium*, 64–5]

49 Celsus, *Prooemium*, 68–75 [attempting to show how he can make some sense out of the many conflicting theories of Hellenistic medicine]. Varro, *On the*

Latin Language, IX, 111, notes the confusion in medical and musical theories, but in IX, 11, uses *medicus* to describe a doctor such as Celsus [the *medicus* deals with the correction of bad habits to keep the patients healthy]. Pliny, XXXIV, 25. 108, is slightly more bitter ['these doctors are ignorant . . . they are well supplied with names']

50 Celsus, *Prooemium*, 23–35, 45–53, 74–5

51 Celsus, VII, prooemium, 1–3 ; V. prooemium. This section dealing with drugs shows Celsus' dependence upon Hellenistic books; here the Roman is not on as sure ground as he is when he speaks of surgery (Celsus, VII) and the book abounds with 'quod Graeci . . . appellant' (V. 1. 1), 'quod . . . Graece dicitur . . .' (V, 4), 'quod . . . a Graecis nominatur' (V, 5), '. . . Graeci vocant' (V, 15), 'quod Graeci habent . . .' (V, 17. 1), and the like. Celsus, *Prooemium*, 1–12, gives a short summary of the development of Greek medicine (of which he says, 'Verum tamen apud Graecos aliquanto magis quam in ceteris nationibus exculta est, *ac ne apud hos quidem a prima origine, sed paucis ante nos saeculis* [*Prooemium*, 2], and then writes (*Prooemium*, 12), 'Et quia prima in eo dissensio est, quod alii sibi experimentorum tantummodo notitiam necessarium esse contendunt, alii nisi corporum rerumque ratione comperta non satis potentum usum esse proponunt, indicandum est, quae maxime ex utraque parte dicantur, quo facilius nostra quoque opinio interponi possit'

52 Celsus makes clear his views of Hellenistic medicine and its intimate joining with philosophy, much to the Roman displeasure (*Prooemium*, 29): 'Etiam sapientiae studiosos maximos medicos esse, si ratiocinatio hoc faceret: nunc illis verba superesse, deesse medendi scientiam.' Celsus understands well that Greek medicine was an integral part of Greek philosophical speculation

53 Vogt, 32–7

54 Celsus, V. 26. 1 C–D: 'In his autem ante omnia scire medicus debet, quae insanabilia sint, quae difficilem curationem habeant, quae promptiorum. . . . Sed ut haec prudenti viro conveniunt, sic rursus histrionis est parvam rem adtollere, quo plus praestitisse videatur'

55 J. Scarborough, 'The Classical Background of the Vesalian Revolution', *Episteme*, II (1968), 200–18

56 Celsus, I, 2. 2

57 *Ibid.*, I, 2. 5. I would differ considerably in translation from Spencer, *LCL*, I, 47, on this passage, and the consequent interpretation

58 Celsus, I, 1. 4

59 This is a transliteration of ὁ ἰατραλείπτης, a physician who cures by the process of anointing, that is an ointment doctor. Pliny, *Letters*, X, 4. 1. Petronius, 28. 3

60 Celsus, I, 1. 1. This passage is parallel to Hippocrates, IV, 346 (*LCL*)

61 Celsus, *Prooemium*, 73–5

62 Celsus mentions only one other Latin writer on medicine, one Cassius, who wrote a Greek medical work and died shortly before Celsus' day. M. Well-

mann, *A. Cornelius Celsus. Eine Quellenuntersuchung* (Berlin, 1913), considers Celsus the copyist of this Cassius, although Wellmann later changed his mind. Spencer, *LCL*, III, 629, confuses this Cassius with an obscure Cassius Iatrosophista who practised in the first decade of the third century. Examples, in Celsus, are numerous on opinions of Hellenistic physicians. I, 4 [Diocles]; I, 6 [Praxagoras]; I, 6-8, 14-16 [Herophilus]. Other names of the Hellenistic tradition are listed in Celsus (*LCL*), III, 628-32

63 A common source, Heracleides of Tarentum, can be seen comparing Celsus, VI, 6. 4, with Galen, XII, 806; Celsus, VI, 18. 8, with Galen, XIII, 831; Celsus V, 18. 6, with Caelius Aurelianus, *Acute Diseases*, II, 24. 136; Celsus, V, 20. 3, with Galen, XIII, 829

64 Celsus, V, *Prooemium*, 2

65 Columella's career in the army in Italy is recorded in *CIL*, IX, 235. His writing was done *c.* 50-65 [Rose, 430]

66 Columella, I, 8. 16. Cato, 56-7

67 Pliny, XX, 33

68 Pliny, *Letters*, VI, 16

69 Pliny, XX, 33. Trans. by J. Bostock, *The Natural History of Pliny* (London, 1856), IV, 235 [BCL]

70 *Ibid.*, 237

71 Stahl, 107

72 L. Kanner, 'Contemporary Folk-Treatment of Sternutation', *BHM*, XI (1942), 273-91

CHAPTER V

1 *Vid.* J. Scarborough, 'Roman Medicine and the Legions: A Reconsideration', *Medical History*, XII (1968), 254-61, with full bibliography. The chapter below is a revised version of the article. To the bibliography of the article should be added the short consideration in J. Harmand, *L'armée et le soldat à Rome* (Paris, 1967), 201-9 (which follows Jacob in general conclusions, but correctly emphasizes the 'sanitary discipline' of the Roman legion); R. G. Penn, 'Medical Services of the Roman Army', *Journal of the Royal Army Medical Corps*, CX (1964), 253-58; E. H. Byrne, 'Medicine in the Roman Army'; *CJ*, V (1909-10), 267-72; and E. Dutoit, 'Tite-Live s'est-il intéressé à la médecine?', *Museum Helveticum*, V (1948), 116-23

2 Dionysius of Halicarnassus, IX, 50. 5 [the description of soldiers putting on themselves fake wound dressings so as to escape fighting; the soldiers were accustomed to put on their own bandages]. Polybius, III, 66. 9 [Publius cares for himself and his wounded]. Plutarch, *Antony*, 43. 1 [Antony gives sympathy to his wounded soldiers; they in turn beg him 'to treat himself']. Plutarch, *Crassus*, 25. 5 [the soldiers are pictured as attempting to pull the barbed Parthian arrows from their own wounds]. So-called Stoicism: O.

Jacob, 'Le service de santé dans les armées Romaines', *L'antiquité classique*, II (1933), 313–29 [317–18]

3 Livy, IV, 39; XXXVII, 33; XL, 33

4 Dionysius of Halicarnassus, IX, 50. 5. Cato, 114–15, 127, 156–60, indicates what sort of 'medicine' was known by the Roman citizen in the Republic, and Roman citizens served in the legions

5 C. Lamarre, *De la milice Romaine* (Paris, 1870), 352, thinks otherwise

6 F. E. Adcock, *The Greek and Macedonian Art of War* (Berkeley, 1962), 14–28, 64–98, and *The Roman Art of War under the Republic* (Cambridge, 1963), 3–28. H. M. D. Parker, *Roman Legions* (Cambridge [rpt.], 1961), 1–46

7 Plutarch, *Marius*, 6. 3; *Caesar*, 34. 3; *Pompey*, 2. 5–6

8 Onasander, *The General*, I, 13–15

9 Onasander, *The General*, VI, 6: Λαμβανέτω δὴ τὴν θεραπείαν καὶ τὰ ὑποζύγια καὶ τὴν ἀποσκευὴν ἅπασαν ἐν μέσῃ τῇ δυνάμει καὶ μὴ χωρίς. Θεραπεία is ambiguous, suggesting a 'preparation of fat for medicinal use' (Dioscorides, II, 76 [ed. M. Wellmann]), a person who 'takes care of the animals' (Aristotle, *Historia Animalium*, 578a7), a substance 'for treatment' (Galen, I, 400), or in a collective sense, simply 'the body of attendants' (Herodotus, I, 199; V, 21; VII, 184). Titchener and Pease [Loeb] translate the idea as 'medical equipment', over-defining the Greek.

10 Onasander, *The General*, I, 14: οἱ μὲν γὰρ ἐκείνους μόνους τοῖς φαρμάκοις θεραπεύουσιν . . . . In Aeneas Tacticus, XXVI, 8–9, θεραπείαν forms a part of formal military vocabulary, rendered as 'careful attention'. D. Barends, *Lexicon Aeneium* (Amsterdam, 1955), 67, and L. W. Hunter, 'Aeneas Tacticus and Stichometry', *CQ*, VII (1913), 256–64

11 Quintus Curtius, *History of Alexander*, IX, 5. 22–5

12 Onasander's work makes no claim to originality, nor to exposition of contemporary problems, but rather it is an attempt to record the traditions of the Hellenistic phalanx in distinction from the Roman legion. Only in one instance, ch. XIX, is a manœuvre suggested which reflects Roman manipular tactics. Onasander's purpose is to outline the qualities required of commanders, which could apply to Hellenistic or Roman generals. W. A. Oldfather in the introduction to the Loeb Onasander, 350

13 Cicero, *Tusculan Disputations*, II, 16. 38

14 Plutarch, *Aemilius Paulus*, 22. 1 [used for celebration for victory]; *Brutus*, 4. 4 [his tent contained refreshment for the tired general]

15 Xenophon, *Anabasis*, III, 4. 30: 'They appointed eight physicians for there were many wounded.' J. Stuart, ed., 'Was the Roman Army Supplied with Medical Officers?', *Archaeological Essays* (Edinburgh, 1872), 197–227 [208], thinks this passage means there were eight soldiers who were trained physicians and who knew surgery

16 Vogt, 46–51 [46]

17 Polybius, III, 66. 9. That a general would 'care for himself and his wounded' indicates that the tradition was strong

18 Cicero, *Tusculan Disputations*, II, 16. 38

19 Silius Italicus, VI, 68–9. Caesar, *African War*, 21

20 *Medicus* as used in Latin literature takes on a variety of meanings. In Silius Italicus, III, 300, it has a definite connotation of magic. In Vergil, *Georgics*, III, 455, and Ovid, *Tristia*, V, 6. 12, the term denotes merely 'healing ability'. Cicero, *Pro Cluentio*, XXI, 57, Suetonius, *Nero*, 37, Plautus, *Menaechmi*, V, 3. 9, and Juvenal, II, 13, use *medicus* to signify what we would term a physician or surgeon. Pliny, XXIX, 6. 13, attempts to define his subject by referring to a 'wound specialist' [*vulnerarius*]

21 Macrobius, *Saturnalia*, I, 17. 15. Vergil, *Aeneid*, XII, 391–7

22 Quintus Smyrnaeus, *Fall of Troy*, IV, 395–405

23 Quintus Smyrnaeus, IV, 538–40

24 Quintus Smyrnaeus, IX, 461–66

25 Quintus Curtius, *History of Alexander*, VI, 10. 34–5. The actual 'evidence' of medical care in the army from Quintus Smyrnaeus or Quintus Curtius, whether from the very ancient Homeric time, Hellenistic days, or even from the contemporary era is highly questionable [Quintus Smyrnaeus, fl. c. AD 390; *vid.* W. F. J. Knight, in *CQ*, XXVI (1932), 178–89; sources: Homer, the 'Cyclical Poets', Proclus, and his own interpretation, along with a common source of Vergil's, one Peisander, as indicated by Macrobius, *Saturnalia*, V, 2. Quintus Curtius Rufus, fl. under Claudius, or Vespasian, and drew his materials from Hellenistic panegyrical sources, as Clitarchus, and possibly from Ptolemy and Aristobulus. *Vid.* E. Schwartz, *PWK*, IV, 1870. Curtius handles his sources with some care, saying (IX, 1. 34; X, 10. 11) he is setting down more than he believes so as not to leave out anything his authorities tell him, but his purpose is rhetorical and dramatic in the Peripatetic model]. It does, however, give us a glimpse at the popular impression of such activity

26 Quintus Curtius, IX, 5. 22–5

27 Quintus Curtius, IX, 5. 25–6

28 Quintus Curtius, IX, 8. 20

29 Vergil, *Aeneid*, XII, 391–7. Trans. C. Day Lewis, *Vergil's Aeneid* (New York, 1953), 301

30 Ennius [ed. Vahlen], frgs. 140, 284, 285, 609

31 Caesar, *Gallic War*, VI, 38. 1–4

32 e.g. *Gallic War*, IV, 12. 4; V, 35. 6

33 *Gallic War*, I, 26. 5; V, 52. 2 and 35. 8; VI, 38. 1–4. Plutarch, *Caesar*, 16

34 Jacob, 326

35 Plutarch, *Crassus* 24–5

36 Plutarch, *Marius*, 6. 3: ἔγνω παρασκεῖν ἑαυτὸν τῷ ἰατρῷ. In *Tiberius Gracchus*, 5. 4, Plutarch notes that camp followers include what are probably medical attendants: ἄνευ θεραπείας καὶ τῶν ἔξω τάξεως ἑπομένων.

37 *Civil War*, III, 78. 2. *African War*, 21

38 Velleius Paterculus, II, 114. 3 [by implication]. Tacitus, *Histories*, II, 45:

'Isdem tentoriis alii fratrem, alii propinquorum fovebant'

39 Caesar, *Civil War*, III, 87. 2

40 Caesar, *Gallic War*, I, 41. 3. Parker, *Roman Legions*, 32

41 Haberling, 26, notices this problem ['. . . trotzdem er (Deciminus: *medicus ordinarius legionis* in Lower Germany [*CIL*, III, 4279]) aktiver Soldat war . . .'], but quickly passes over it to other matters. Haberling's study has a magnificent summary 'proving' that physicians were in the legions.

The informal status of the title is firmly indicated by the multiplicity of designations of the *medici* in the legions. *CIL*, XIII, 7943 [M. Sabinianus Quictus, *medicus miles* of the I Minervia at Bonn]. *CIL*, III, 14347⁵ [T. Aurelius Numerius, *medicus legionis* of the XXII Primigenia from Aquincum in Hungary]. *CIL*, III, 5959 [Ulpius Lucilianus, *medicus ordinarius* of the III Italica from Lambaesis in Algeria]. *CIL*, III, 6532 [an anonymous *medicus*(?) *ordinarius legionis* of the III Italica from Castra Regina (Regensberg)]. *CIL*, VIII, 18314 [Papirius Aelianus, *medicus ordinarius legionis* of the III Augusta from Lambaesis]. *CIL*, III, 3413 [Marcus Marcellus, *medicus* of an undetermined legion from Aquincum]. This inscription is an important one, clearly showing the status of the *medicus* and how the probable system functioned under the direction of a superior officer: 'Asclepio et Hygiae Mar(cius) Marcellus, med(icus) sub c(ur)a(gente?) P. Va[l(erio)] Praesent(e) evoc(ato) v(otum) s(olvit) l(ibens) m(erito).' *CIL*, III, 14349⁷ [Caius Nundinius Optervius, *medicus stipendiis* of an undetermined legion from Aquincum]. Greek inscriptions tell another side of the story. *IGRR*, I. 1212, shows a Greek physician functioning in the II Trajana from Thebae in Egypt [dated AD 147]. *IGRR*, I. 1361 [*OGIS*, 207], indicates that an Egyptian temple physician was servicing the XXII Deiotariana in the Hellenistic tradition. In the Latin inscriptions other titles abound. *CIL*, VI, 2532 [Rome]: *medicus clinicis cohortis*. *CIL*, XIII, 1833 [Lugdunum]: *medicus castrensis*, are but two of many varieties

42 *CIL*, VII, 690

43 The individuals who function as *medici* in the auxilia show their non-Roman origins [names listed in Haberling, 73], but their designations follow the pattern noted for the legions. E.g. *CIL*, III, 4279, 5959, 6532; XIII, 6621, 7094, 7415

44 *CIL*, XIII, 2308

45 *CIL*, VI, 2532

46 *CIL*, VI, 3910; VII, 1144; X, 3442–4; XI, 19. A. von Domaszewski, *Die Rangordnung des römischen Heeres* (Bonn, 1908), 15 and 45. C. G. Starr, *Roman Imperial Navy* (Cambridge, 1960), 56. *Duplicarius* merely indicates that the individual received double pay. G. T. Haneveld, 'Medical Service with the Roman Fleet' (in Dutch), *Ned. milit. geneesk.*, XVIII (1965), 288–90

47 The literature on the legionary hospitals is plentiful. Examples are I. A. Richmond, 'Roman Britain and Roman Military Antiquities', *Proceedings of the British Academy*, XLI (1955), 297–315 [314–15]; R. Schultze, 'Die

römische Legionslazarette in Vetera und anderen Legionslagern', *Bonner Jahrbücher*, CXXXIX (1934), 54–63; and C. Koenen, 'Beschreibung von Novaesium', *Bonner Jahrbücher*, CXI–CXII (1904), 97–242 [5–6, 28, 53–4, 180–2]

48 Richmond, 314–15. Schultze, 56–8

49 Velleius Paterculus, II, 114. 1–3. Trans. F. W. Shipley (Loeb)

50 Tacitus, *Annals*, I, 69

51 Tacitus, *Histories*, II, 45

52 Celsus, *Prooemium*, 43. Galen, XIII, 604

53 Celsus, VII, 5

54 In another context, Galen gives a clue to the regard within the legion for the *medicus*. In quoting from the 'military physician' Antigonus, Galen begins as follows [XII, 557]: "Ἄλλο Ἀντιγόνου ἐν στρατοπέδῳ ἐπισήμως ἰατρεύσαντος. The key is the use of ἐπισήμως, which in this context can be rendered as 'approved', or 'designated', or 'marked off as'. Approval is indicated with the use of ἐπίσημος by Isocrates, XII, 2 [ed. Blass]. Polybius, I, 37. 4, uses ἐπισημασία to tell of an 'appearance' and the same use is found in Plutarch, *Numa*, 22, and *Sulla*, 14. Galen, XIV, 661, uses the root in a passive sense 'showing' symptoms of a disease, as does Thucydides, II, 49: τῶν ἀκρωτηρίων ἀντίληψις αὐτοῦ ἐπεσήμαινειν ['The seizure of his extremities set a mark upon him' (Liddell and Scott, 655)]. Thus our original passage from Galen [XII, 557] should be rendered something like 'Another [recipe] of Antigonus, designated as practising medicine in a legionary camp'. This evidence links well with the inscriptional story of the 'designation' of the *medicus*

55 K. Lehmann-Hartleben, *Die Traianssäule* (Berlin, 1926), plate 22 [XL–XLI]. Useful is I. A. Richmond, 'Trajan's Army on Trajan's Column', *Papers of the British School at Rome*, XIII (1935), 1–40 [13–14]

56 Lehmann-Hartleben, plate 22. The soldiers being treated are looking at the *medici* with pained resignation

57 *SHA, Aurelian*, VII, 8

58 *Ibid.*

59 Vegetius, III, 2. In II, 10, Vegetius describes how medical care is seen to by the praefect of the camp, and this is what the evidence of *CIL*, III, 3413 would indicate [inscription quoted in note 41 above]

60 Lucian, *Gout*, is an example of a bitter caricature of the helpless doctor with many promises

61 Galen, XIV, 649–50

CHAPTER VI

1 A. Söllner, *Die hygienischen Anschauungen des römischen Architekten Vitruvius* (Jena, 1913)

2 G. E. Gask and J. Todd, 'The Origins of Hospitals', *SMH*, I, 122–30 (123). Celsus, *Prooemium*, 65. Columella, XII, 1. 6; XII, 3. 7–8

3 Varro, I, 13. Vitruvius, I, 4. Columella, I. 5

4 The best collection of plates and references is Milne. Other useful references for illustrations of medical tools are *Instruments de chirurgie Gréco-Romains* (Geneva, 1961); R. Caton and W. H. Buckler, 'Medical and Surgical Instruments found at Kolophon', *PRS*, VII (1914), 235–42; R. Caton, 'Medical and Surgical Instruments found near Colophon', *JHS*, XXXIV (1914), 114–18 and plates X–XIII; and B. Vulpes, *Illustrazione di tutti gli instrumenti chirurgici scavati in Ercolano e in Pompei* (Naples, 1847), which is a collection of articles and references published previously by Vulpes and Quaranta, and forms the basis of Milne. *Cf.* T. Meyer-Steineg, *Chirurgische Instrumente des Altertums* (Jena, 1912), and J. Como, 'Das Grab eines römischen Arztes bei Bingen', *Germania*, IX (1925), 152–62

5 Vitruvius, VIII, 3 and 4. Cicero, *On Divination*, II 123. Frontinus, *Aqueducts*, prologue, 1 Varro, I, 13

6 Celsus, *Prooemium*. Frontinus, *Aqueducts*, II, 93

7 Gask and Todd, *SMH*, I, 123–4

8 *Cf.* note 47, chapter V above. Gask and Todd, *SMH*, I, 122–3. D. R. Wilson, 199–220 (esp. 199 with fig. 10, p. 200). B. Fricker, *Ein römischer Militärspital* (Zurich, 1898), C. Brunner, *Die Spuren der römischen Aerzte in der Schweiz* (Zurich, 1894), and F. Stähelin, *Die Schweiz in römischer Zeit* (Basel, 1927), 416–21, summarize the finds in Switzerland. *Cf. CIL*, XIII, 5079, 5208, 5053, 5277, 10021, and 10027

9 Richmond, 313–15. Some inscriptions may indicate 'hospital directions' (*ad valetudinarium; a valetudinario*). *CIL*, VI, 4475, 8639; X, 6637

10 Richmond, 315

11 Wilson, 199, 204, 207–8, 211, 215, 220

12 *Cf.* note 8 above (Switzerland) and note 47, chapter V above (Germany). K. H. Knoerzer, 'Römerzeitliche Heilkräuter aus Novaesium', *AGM*, XLIX (1965), 416–22, notes plants used in drug-making, as does his article 'Ein Beispiel für die Anwendung phytosoziologischer Kenntnisse bei der Grabungsforschung'. *Bonner Jahrbücher*, LXIII (1963), 260–5. For recent work related to the German hospital systems, *vid.* A. Stieren, 'Die neuen Grabungen in Haltern', *Germania*, XII (1928), 70–6; F. Oelmann, 'Ausgrabungen in Vetera 1930', *Germania*, XV (1931), 221–9; and P. Jetter, *Geschichte des Hospitals* (Wiesbaden, 1966: Supp. *AGM*, No. 5), 1–8 (good diagrams, pp. 2–5). V. L. Bologa and V. Manoliu, 'Medizin-historisches aus dem römischen Dazien', *AGM*, XLVIII (1964), 289–98 (Rumania). V.

Bazala, 'Le istituzioni mediche romane nelle odierne regioni croate', *Pag. Storia Med.*, XI (1967), 10–24 (Croatia)

13 M. Wheeler, *Roman Art and Architecture* (London, 1964), 108. R. G. Good-child and J. B. Ward-Perkins, 'The Limes Tripolitanus in the Light of Recent Discoveries', *JRS*, XXXIX (1949), 81–95, 'Roman Sites on the Tarhuna Plateau of Tripolitania', *Papers of the British School at Rome*, XIX (1951), 43–77, and 'Roman Tripolitania: Reconnaissance in the Desert Frontier Zone', *The Geographical Journal*, CXV (1950), 161–78. J. B. Ward-Perkins and J. M. C. Toynbee, 'The Hunting Baths at Lepcis Magna,' *Archaeologia*, XCIII (1949), 165–95. P. Romanelli, 'La Prima Linea di Difesa di Leptis Magna', *Archaeologia Classica*, IV (1952), 100–2.

14 Celsus, *Prooemium*, 65: 'Et qui ampla valetudinaria nutriunt. . . .' This is rendered by Spencer [*LCL*, I, 35] as 'those who take charge of large hospitals . . .', which cannot be correct if one compares the references to *valetudinaria* found in Columella, XI, 1. 18; XII, 1. 6. A better translation would be something akin to a 'large sick-bay' or 'roomy sick-room'.

15 This seems to be the meaning of Celsus, *Prooemium*, 65: '. . . quia singulis summa cura consulere non sustinent, ad communia ista confugiunt.' The context firmly shows the Roman *pater familias* as the chief participant and director of the facilities for the comfort of the sick in his household. This is in keeping with the customary procedure noted in Cato, I, 1 and 2, and in Columella, XI, 1. 18; XII, 1. 6, and 3. 7–8

16 Mathhew, XXV, 36

17 Justin Martyr, *First Apology*, I, 67

18 Julian, *Letters*, XXII, 430 [*LCL*, III, 68–9]

19 Gask and Todd, *SMH.*, I, 129–30

20 Vitruvius, V., 9. Leake, *AMH*, II (1930), 140

21 Wheeler, *Roman Art and Architecture*, 106–10. D. Krencker, *Die Trierer Kaiserthermen* (Augsburg, 1929). F. Brown, *Roman Architecture* (New York, 1965), 38, 23–4, with plates 72–3, 33, 74–5. E. D. Thatcher, 'The Open Rooms of the Terme del Foro at Ostia', *Memoirs of the American Academy in Rome*, XXIV (1956), 167–264. P. MacKendrick, *The Mute Stones Speak* (New York, 1960), 137, 189, 296–9, 309, 319 [the baths at Rome] with references. Jules Rouyer, *Études médicales sur l'ancienne Rome* (Paris, 1859), 1–31. G. Pinto, *Storia della medicina in Roma* (Rome, 1879). Andre Palladio, *Les thermes des Romains* (Paris, 1838). W. J. Anderson, R. P. Spiers, and T. Ashby, *The Architecture of Ancient Rome* (London, 1927), ch. VI, is the best summary of the material from Rome.

22 Horace, *Satires*, I, 4. 71–4. Petronius, 91–2. Vitruvius, V, 10

23 H. Drerup, 'Architektur als Symbol', *Gymnasium*, LXXIII (1966), 181–96, with plates I–VIII. Pliny, XXXVI, 101.

24 P. H. Futcher, 'Notes on Insect Contagion', *BHM*, IV (1936), 536–58, assumes 'scientific insight' on the part of the Romans.

25 Varro, I, 12. Trans. W. D. Hooper [*LCL*, 209]

26 Varro, I, 12. Trans. Hooper [*LCL*, 209–10]
27 Columella, I, 5
28 Cato, V
29 *SEHRE*, I, 203–5, 225–8
30 Celsus, VII, prooemium. Galen, II, 272
31 R. J. Forbes, *Metallurgy in Antiquity* (Leiden, 1950). E. H. Schulz, 'Zur Frage der Entwicklung des Stahles für ärztliche Instrumente', *AGM*, XXXIX (1955), 30–4. F. Kudlien, 'Wissenschaftlicher und instrumenteller Fortschritt in ihrer Wechselwirkung in der antiken Chirurgie', *AGM*, XLV (1961), 329–33
32 Knoerzer's articles in note 12 above. J. M. Riddle, 'The Introduction and Use of Eastern Drugs in the Early Middle Ages', *AGM*, XLIX (1965) 185–98, indicates that matters were similar later. Cicero, *On Duties*, I, 42. 150 Horace, *Satires*, II, 3. 228; *CIL*, I, 1062 (*unguentarii*). Scribonius Largus, 22; *Digest*, XLVIII, 8. 3. 3 (*pigmentarii*). *CIL*, VI, 384 (*aromatarius*). Generally *vid.* A. Schmidt, *Drogen und Drogenhandel im Altertum* (Leipzig, 1924), H. O. Lenz, *Botanik der alten Griechen und Romer* (Gotha, 1859), and Schmidt in *PWK*, suppl. V, 172–82. Galen shows his knowledge of surface anatomy in his dissection of the forearm (II, 272–9), and he performs well on what appears to be a Rhesus monkey
33 Celsus, VII, 5. 3. Milne, 142
34 Milne, plate XLV, fig. 4
35 Galen, XIV, 787
36 Catheters: Celsus, VII, 26. Paul of Aegina, VI, 19. Specimens of both male and female catheters from the House of the Surgeon in Pompeii can be seen in the Naples Museum. Figs 7, 8 and 9 are based upon Milne, plate XLV, figs 1 and 2. Forceps: Galen, X, 450. Milne, 135
37 Milne, 135
38 Galen, XII, 622. Celsus, VI, 7. 1. Scribonius Largus, 39. Marcellus Empiricus, IX, 1
39 Galen, XII, 623
40 Milne has many references to various finds throughout Europe, particularly in connection with the many military *valetudinaria*. G. Calza, *La Necropoli del Porto di Roma nell' Isola Sacra* (Rome, 1940), 257 and fig. 150, provides an example of actual manufacture of surgical tools in the Empire. A blacksmith and his forge are pictured, along with a remarkable variety of instruments and tools that he has produced. Hatchets, hammers, kitchen knives, saws, metal-cutters are represented along with what appears to be a box of surgical scalpels [from Ostia]. Calza, 250, and fig. 149, shows a more elaborate set of tools and their use [bleeding a patient's leg], but their form is essentially akin to those from the blacksmith's shop. Both illustrations are reproduced in *SEHRE*, I, plate XXXII, fig. 1, and plate XXXI, fig. 1
41 Milne, 144–5 [Germany], 147 [Athens], 169 [Brussels], 34 [Rome], 35 [Wroxeter], and numerous references to Naples and Pompeii

42 A. Maiuri, *Pompei* (Naples, n. d.), 69–71. R. C. Bell, 'A Surgeon of Pompeii', *British Journal of Plastic Surgery*, XII (1959), 177–82

43 Galen, XIII, 604

44 *Ibid.*, II, 682

45 Milne, 12

46 *Ibid.* O. Davies, *Roman Mines in Europe* (Oxford, 1935)

47 Hippocrates, I, 58

48 Scribonius Largus, 37

49 *Ibid.* Marcellus Empiricus, XIV, 44

50 Hippocrates, III, 174

51 Gold cautery: Theodorus Priscianus, *Logicus*, 22. Tin: Scribonius Largus, 268. Milne, 15, describes a tin weight for medicines housed in the Museum at Chester

52 Milne, 16

53 Scribonius Largus, 83

54 Milne, 17

55 Hippocrates, III, 331. Scribonius Largus, 7. Galen, XI, 125. Recent studies (from France and England) further bear out a surprising level of sophistication. M. A. Dollfuss, 'L'Étonnante Instrumentation des Opthalmologistes Gallo-Romains', *Archeologia*, X (1966) 16–19 [*cf.* C. L. Grotefend, *Die Stempel der römischen Augenärzte* (Hanover, 1867], and C. Wells, 'A Roman Surgical Instrument from Norfolk', *Antiquity*, XLI (1967), 139–41

56 F. H. Garrison, 'The History of Drainage, Irrigation, Sewage Disposal, and Water-Supply', *Bulletin of the New York Academy of Medicine*, V (1929), 887–938 [894]

57 Livy, I, 56. A. Alföldi, *Early Rome and the Latins* (Ann Arbor, 1965), 133, 195, 198, with references

58 Pliny, XXXVI, 24

59 *Ibid.*, XXXI, 1–34

60 Seneca, *Epistulae*, 86. 6–7. Not all citizens were enthusiastic. Athenaeus, I, 18c quotes a certain Antiphanes, who says, 'To hell with the bath! It has put me in a miserable state. I am now a piece of boiled meat. Anybody could grab me, taking a grasp of my skin and scrape it off. Hot water is a cruel thing.' *Cf.* Petronius, *Sat.*, 42

61 Frontinus, *Aqueducts*, Prologue; II, 87–91

62 Vitruvius, I, 4. 2–5

63 Vitruvius, VIII, 3. 28–4. 1. This and the preceding passage [I, 4. 1–7] translated by M. H. Morgan, *Vitruvius: the Ten Books on Architecture* (Dover Reprint, New York, 1960)

64 Vitruvius, VIII, 1. Frontinus, *Aqueducts*, II, 93

65 T. Ashby, *Aqueducts of Ancient Rome* (Oxford, 1935). Frontinus' description is one of nine aqueducts built up to his day. They are: Aqua Appia [312 BC], Anio Vetus [272–269 BC], Aqua Marcia [146 BC], Aqua Tepula [125 BC], Aqua Julia [33 BC], Aqua Virgo [33–19 BC], Aqua Alsientia [AD 10], Aqua

Claudia [38–52], and the Aqua Nova [38–52]
66 Frontinus, *Aqueducts*, prologue, 1
67 *Ibid.*, II, 88
68 *Ibid.*, I, 33–7; I, 19
69 Frontinus, *Aqueducts*, I, 4–23. Vitruvius, VIII, 6. Pliny, XXXI, 57. Generally, E. B. van Deman, *The Building of Roman Aqueducts* (Washington, 1943)
70 Vegetius, 3, 2

CHAPTER VII

1 E. F. Cordell, 'The Medicine and Doctors of Horace', *JHB*, XII (1901), 233–40 [237–8]
2 Horace, *Satires*, I, 2. 1
3 Horace, *Odes*, III, 22. 2
4 Horace, *Epistulae*, II, 1. 114. Quoted in Cordell, 235, from the metrical translation of Sir Theodore Martin
5 My translation may overdefine the meaning. S. P. Bovie, *Satires and Epistles of Horace* (Chicago, 1963), 207, interprets the line as 'Their wounds only fools conceal: the wise let them heal', which would put the physician completely out of consideration. Horace, *Epistulae*, I, 16. 24
6 E. Fraenkel, *Horace* (Oxford, 1966), 444
7 *Ibid.*, 265–73
8 Horace, *Odes*, II, 3
9 Horace, *Satires*, I, 2. 1–7. Martial, IX, 96
10 Martial, VI, 31. Anonymous translation, *BCL*, 275
11 Seneca, *On Benefits*, VI, 15. 2
12 *Ibid.*, VI, 16. 1
13 *Ibid.*, VI, 15. 1
14 *Ibid.*, VI, 16. 3
15 Suetonius, *Caesar*, 42 [citizenship to doctors in Rome]; *Augustus*, 42 [foreign residents expelled excepting doctors, teachers, and a large number of household slaves]: *Augustus*, 81 [much unsuccessful treatment of Augustus' ills until Antonius Musa's 'cold baths, which countered all medical practice'; *Tiberius*, 72 [Tiberius' suspicion of his doctor Charicles]. Cassius Dio, LIII, 30. 3 [Augustus grants civic immunity to physicians in Rome after Musa cures him]; LIII, 30. 4–5 [Musa treats Marcellus but fails]
16 Pliny, XXIX, 1, 6, and 8. *CIL*, VI, 9562–617, would seem to bear this out. Freedmen Greek physicians established themselves in Gaul, and Pliny bitterly notes how much money they made (Pliny, XXIX, 5. 9–10 and 8. 22). Individual physicians did occasionally command great respect, but not for their medical art (*CIL*, XI, 5399–400 [from Asisium in Italy] praises a doctor for his civic-mindedness in contributing 37,000 sesterces for paving a public road)

17 Tacitus, *Annals*, XII, 61

18 Tacitus, *Annals*, XII, 67. 2

19 The letter begins, 'Germano Claudio regi et deo aeterno', A. Momigliano, *Claudius* (Cambridge, 1961), 91. The Latin version of the letter is given by F. Cumont in *Revue Philologique*, XLII (1918), 85 ff. *Cf.* K. Deichgräber, 'Professio Medici: zum Vorwort Scribonius Largus', *Abhandlungen Akademie Mainz*, IX (1950), 853–79

20 Momigliano, *Claudius*, 28, 91–2, and 'Una lettera a Claudio e una lettera ad Antigono Gonato', *Athenaeum*, XI (1933), 128–42. Nero had some of this uncritical cultural omnivorousness in his relation with his physician Andromachus (Galen, XIV, 2). From time to time, Celsus exhibits this characteristic, though guardedly. V, 26. 31: 'Id genus a Graecis diductum in species est, nostris vocabulis non est'

21 Tactitus, *Histories*, IV, 81

22 K. Wellesley, trans., *Tacitus: The Histories* (Baltimore, 1964), 263–4, captures the Tacitean irony well: '. . . this fellow threw himself at Vespasian's feet, imploring him, with groans, to heal his blindness. He had been told to make his request by Serapis, the favourite god of a nation much addicted to strange beliefs. . . . a second petitioner, who suffered a withered hand, pleaded his case too. . . . Would Caesar tread upon him with the royal foot? . . . With a smiling expression, and surrounded by an expectant crowd of bystanders, he did what was asked. Instantly the cripple recovered the use of his hand, and the light of day dawned again upon his blind companion. Both these incidents are vouched for by eye-witnesses, though there is nothing now to be gained by lying.' *Histories*, IV, 81. 2

23 Wellesley, trans., *Histories*, 263. *Cf.* R. Syme, *Tacitus* (Oxford, 1957), I, 206

24 *Greek Anthology*, XI, 113 [Nicarchus]. W. R. Paton, trans., *LCL*, IV, 125

25 *Ibid.*, 118 [*LCL*, IV, 127]. (Callicter)

26 *Ibid.*, 122 [*LCL*, IV, 129]. (Callicter)

27 *Ibid.*, 120 [*LCL*, IV, 129]. (Callicter). Other caustic inscriptions, poems, and epigrams relating to doctors are found in the *Greek Anthology* [*LCL*], IV, Book XI, 112–26, 257, 280–1, 382, 401

28 Pliny, XXV, 197. Galen, XIII, 636–8

29 Pausanias, X, 32. 1

30 Pliny, XXXIV, 108

31 Gargilius Martialis, *Preface*, 7 (ed. Rose)

32 Scribonius Largus, *Preface*

33 Galen, XV, 313–16

34 Epictetus, III, 23. 30

35 Epictetus, III, 23. 27

36 Dioscorides, II, 36. Galen, XII, 216–17

37 Galen, XII, 248–50, 423–4, 772; XIII, 703–4, 861

38 *CIL*, XIII, 579 and 1906. Dioscorides, V, 113. Pliny, XXV, 19. 60

39 Pliny, XXXIV, 108

40 Dio Chrysostom, *Discourses*, XXXIII, 6. Trans. J. W. Cohoon and H. L. Crosby, *LCL*, III, 279

41 Lucian, *Remarks to an Illiterate Book Fancier*, 29

42 Plutarch, *How to Tell a Flatterer from a Friend*, 71A (32)

43 Galen, XIV, 600–1

44 Galen, XIV, 600

45 B. P. Grenfell and A. S. Hunt, *The Oxyrhynchus Papyri* (London, 1898), Vol. I, XL, 4–10. Trans. Grenfell and Hunt

46 Grenfell and Hunt, *Oxyrhynchus Papyri*, I, XL, 51–2. S. Eitrem, ed., *Papyri Osloensis*, Fasc. 1, *Magical Papyri* (Oslo, 1925), I, 320–4. J. Lindsay, *Daily Life in Roman Egypt* (London, 1963), 221–8

47 *CIL*, XIII, 5708

48 Caesar, *Gallic War*, VI, 21

49 Celsus, VII, prooemium, 1–2

50 Abortion: Plutarch, *Introduction to Health*, 134. F. R. Hähnel, 'Der künstliche Abortus im Altertum', *AGM*, XXIX (1936), 224–55. That infanticide was practised by the rich is shown by Suetonius, *Augustus*, 65, and *Claudius*, 27; Longus, *Pastoralia*, IV, 35; and Tertullian, *Apologia*, IX. *Cf*. M. Käser, *Das römische Privatrecht* (Munich, 1959), II, 141–5. Hopkins, 136.

   Contraception: N. B. Himes, *A Medical History of Contraception* (London, 1936), 74–98. P. Diepgen, *Die Frauenheilkunde der alten Welt* (Munich, 1937). The problem is hotly argued, as seen in R. Syme, 'Bastards in the Roman Aristocracy', *Proceedings of the American Philosophical Society*, CIV (1960), 324. Hopkins, 129–30, 132–4 (refs for contraception). Antonius Liberalis, *Metamorphoses*, 41 (ed. E. Martin, in *Mythographi Graeci*, II, 124–5), seems to indicate a condom made from a goat's bladder. Himes, 186–8. P. Richter, 'Beiträge zur Geschichte des Kondoms', *Zeitschrift für Bekämpfung der Geschlechtskrankheiten*, XII (1912), 35. K. Hopkins, 'A Textual Emendation in a Fragment of Musonius Rufus', *CQ*, XV (1965), 72–4, offers conclusive proof of contraception among the Romans (the translated fragment is reproduced in Hopkins, 141)

51 Suetonius, *Augustus*, 34 and 39. *CIL*, XI, 6538. *Digest*, XXXV, 1. 64. 1. Constantine formally abolished the laws. *Codex Theod.*, VIII, 16; IX, 42. 9

52 Aristotle, *Historia Animalia*, 583a. Hippocrates (Littré), VII, 490

53 Hopkins, 126, uses comparisons with modern Japan and India. A. Hasanat, *Controlled Parenthood* (Dacca, India, 1945), 103–15, and I. B. Taeuber, *The Population of Japan* (Princeton, 1958), 270–2

54 Hopkins, 126. K. Hopkins, 'The Age of Roman Girls at Marriage', *Population Studies*, XVIII (1965), 325. For his calculations, Hopkins uses UN model life tables, level ten, with an expectation of life at birth for both sexes of 25 (*Methods for Population Projections by Sex and Age*, *UN Population Studies*, XXV (1956), 74–6, ST/SOA/Series A). His median duration of first marriages, with no account taken of divorce, but only of one or both the partners' death, is based 'for purposes of illustration' on a couple married at 15

O

(female) and 25 (male). Although I was unable to obtain it, Hopkins' *A Demographic Profile of the Later Roman Aristocracy* (Unpublished Fellowship Dissertation, King's College, Cambridge, 1963) appears to be helpful in these problems, as is H. Nordberg, *Biometrical Notes* (Helsinki, 1963), which considers Christian inscriptions from Rome. The bibliography on demographics for Roman times increases. Among the more useful are W. R. MacDonell, 'On the Expectation of Life in Ancient Rome, and in the Provinces of Hispania and Lusitania and Africa', *Biometrika*, IX (1913), 366–80; A. R. Burn, 'Hic breve vivitur. A Study of the Expectation of Life in the Roman Empire', *Past and Present*, IV (1953), 1–31; H. Hombert and C. Préaux, 'Note sur la durée de la vie dans l'Égypte gréco-romain', *CE*, XX (1945), 139–46; and L. Moretti, 'Statistica demografia ed epigrafia: Durata media della vita in Roma imperiale', *Epigrafica*, XXI (1959), 60–78. Hopkins, 126–7, rejects 'low fertility' theories as given in O. Seeck, *Geschichte des Untergangs der antiken Welt* (Stuttgart, 1921), IV, 1269–71, and H. Last, 'Letter to N. H. Baynes', *JRS*, XXXVII (1947), 152–6

55 H. Herter, 'Die Soziologie der antiken Prostitution', *Jahrbuch für Antike und Christentum*, III (1960), 70ff. Hopkins, 127

56 Hopkins, 128. *Codex Theod.*, XIII, 3. 9. *CIL*, VI, 9566

57 Pliny, XXIV, 11. 18: 'Tradition tells us of a marvel: that to rub (cedar gum) all over the penis before coitus prevents conception.' (Portentum est quod tradunt abortivum fieri in venere ante perfusa virilitate.) The English places too much stricture on the Latin meaning. It is possible 'prevention of premature birth' is meant. Dioscorides, V, 106. 6 (using alum)

58 Soranus, *Gynecology*, I, 61 (Temkin, 63–4). Dioscorides, II, 159. 3 (contraceptive)

59 Plutarch, *Instruction in Health*, 122 B–F, 129 D, 135 A ('Advice About Keeping Well', *LCL*, Plutarch's *Moralia*, II, 217ff)

60 Plutarch, *Whether the Affections of the Soul are Worse than those of the Body*, 500 E

61 P. A. Stadter, *Plutarch's Historical Methods* (Cambridge, Mass., 1965), 10. Galen, IV, 767. Plutarch mentions a common-knowledge fact in his *Causes of Natural Phenomena*, I. 911 E (fresh water on ashes gives lye) which appears in Galen, XI, 630 (sea and lye compared). Plutarch occasionally cites this physician or that, as he speaks of medical theories, as in *Natural Phenomena*, III, 912 D [Apollonius, a pupil of the Herophilean methods, on digestion in various individuals with differing body types]. Ancient reducing fads prove to be as fascinating as Plutarch rambles along. He says since dew has a natural erosive property about it, one can use it for reducing; at least fat women *think* that dew-soaked clothes or woollens will melt excess fat away [*Natural Phenomena*, VI, 913 F]. His source, or perhaps again common-knowledge, speaks of how dew can erode the skin where the blood supply is not thick [*Natural Phenomena*, VI, 913 E], and is very similar to Pliny *Natural History*, XXXI, 33, and Seneca, *Questiones Naturales*, III, 25, 4, who

say dew causes scabs. Mnesithius of Athens' work on foods is borrowed as Plutarch notes the shrewd physician able to predict diseases from what the patient most wants to eat [*Natural Phenomena*, XXVI, 918 E]. Physicians dish out strong drugs for small hurts, and Plutarch quotes Philotimus' comparison of a sore finger and ulcerated liver [*How to Tell a Flatterer from a Friend*, 73 A–B]. Other references are numerous, but become repetitive of one another.

62 Plutarch's 'scientific vocabulary' is a moot point. Πέψις or πέττειν, adapted by Aristotle from medical writers [*Parts of Animals*, 670a 20ff: the stomach, liver and spleen help in the 'concoction' of the nourishment. But *cf. Generation of Animals*, 715b 24 and 743a 31, where πέττειν is used for the ripening of fruits of plants and the semen of animals], appears in Plutarch, *Causes of Natural Phenomena*, III, 913 A, XXVI, 918 E, as does περίτωμα, which is the 'residue' or 'remainder' of concoction, when the whole product does not assume a converted or assimilable state [Aristotle, *Generation of Animals*, 751b 1 and 739a 2] as in Plutarch, *Natural Phenomena*, XXI, 917 B and XXX, 919 C. Κρᾶσις appears at numerous points in the *Natural Phenomena*. Problems come when the modern translator must determine the exact shading of such a term from the Greek according to context. Galen, I, 509ff, devotes an essay to explaining the concepts current in his day of κρᾶσις with variants of meaning. Thus Plutarch's κρᾶσις in *Natural Phenomena*, IV, 913 A, is 'temperature', or a 'blending of heat and cold'; XVI, 915 E, 'blending'; but in XXXI, 919 D, the literal 'mixture', and so on. All these words are common in Greek, and the modern English reader should be on his guard against the assumption of a strictly 'scientific' vocabulary that would serve a technical need in or out of context. *Vid.* the remarks of F. H. Sandbach in *LCL, Plutarch's Moralia*, XI, 138–41; D. L. Page, 'Thucydides' Description of the Great Plague at Athens', *CQ*, XLVII (1953), 97–120, discusses the same problem with Thucydides vis-à-vis Hippocrates

63 Statius, *Silvae*, I, 4. 98–131

64 Statius, *Silvae*, III, 5. 37–42

65 Statius, *Silvae*, V, 5. 42–3

66 Marcus Cornelius Fronto, *Correspondence*, I, 38, 184, 192, 198, 200, 218 [refs. to *LCL*, vol. and page]

67 Fronto, I, 224, 226, 228

68 Fronto, I, 240, 242

69 Fronto, I, 246, 248, 250

70 Fronto, I, 252, 306, 308; II, 44

71 Fronto, II, 84–6

72 Fronto, II, 88, 152, 156

73 Fronto, II, 174

74 Fronto, II, 232, 242, 252

75 E. R. Dodds, *Pagan and Christian in an Age of Anxiety* (Cambridge, 1965), 40. C. A. Behr, *Aelius Aristides* (Amsterdam, 1968), 12

76 A. J. Festugière, *Personal Religion Among the Greeks* (Berkeley, 1960), 86, says, 'fundamentally he did not want to be cured. To be cured would mean no longer to enjoy the presence and companionship of the god; and precisely what the patient needs is the companionship of the god'

77 Aelius Aristides [ed. Keil], 47. 2–3

78 Aristides, 47. 3–4

79 Dodds, *Anxiety*, 41

80 Aristides, 48. 6 and 57 and 62 [asthma], 49. 17 [hypertension], 48. 57 [head-aches], 47. 5 and 48. 58 [insomnia], 47. 8, 21, 32, 40 and 53; 49. 1. 8; 50. 38 [stomach problems]; 47. 59–60, 73; 48. 42–3, 62–3 [intestinal disorders]

81 Aristides, 47. 8 [calculi]; 49. 11 and 14 [tuberculosis]; 47. 61–8 [prostate problems, but in men under fifty years, this is extremely rare. The description of his problem here includes the growth and recession of a tumour, or something Aristides thought was a tumour. The urethra, bladder, or ureters could have been all involved, according to the rambling account]; 48. 38–45 [typhoid; Aristides describes a plague]; 48. 69; 49. 30 [rhinitis, or something approaching a mixture of hay fever, bronchitis, and a continual common cold]

82 Aristides, 49. 11–12, 16–20 [tetanus; but many of the characteristics of his attack also enter into an epileptic seizure; however, since this series of symptoms appears only twice in Aristides' account, tetanus is a more reasonable conclusion, accompanied, as Aristides says, by a rigidity of his jaws and a stiffness of his face [49. 11]

83 Dodds, *Anxiety*, 41

84 Aristides, 47. 61–8

85 Aristides, 47. 73

86 Aristides, 47. 76–7

87 Aristides, 48. 6

88 Aristides, 48. 20–2

89 Aristides, 48. 21–2

90 Aristides, 48. 34

91 Aristides, 48. 44

92 Aristides, 47–9

93 Aristides, 47. 63–4

94 Aristides, 47. 69

95 Dodds, *Anxiety*, 43, with note 3

96 Galen, XVI, 222

97 Dodds, *Anxiety*, 45, and note 4 (Eitrem)

98 Herzog, 972

99 Galen, X, 4

CHAPTER VIII

1 Suetonius, *Caesar*, 42; *Augustus*, 42
2 Below, 30 [granting of civic immunities]. *CIL*, VI, 4416. *cf.* R. Bozzoni, *I medici ed il diritto romano* (Naples, 1904), 177–81, and I. Fischer, *Ärztliche Standespflichten und Standesfragen* (Leipzig, 1912), 162. Herzog, 1001 [right to form corporations]
3 Vogt, 46–7
4 Pliny, XXIX, 6. 12–13: '. . . eique ius Quiritium datum et tabernam in compito Acilio emptam ob id publice'
5 Pliny, XXIX, 6–8
6 Celsus, *Prooemium*, 27–35, 45–53, 68–75
7 Vogt, 46 and 49
8 Galen, XIV, 599: ἀφ' οὗ γὰρ οἱ τὸ δοκεῖν μᾶλλον ἢ εἶναι σπουδάσαντες οὐ κατὰ τὴν ἰατρικὴν μόνον, ἀλλὰ καὶ τὰς ἄλλας τέχνας ἐπλεόνασαν . . . . Earlier in the treatise, Galen comments that this kind of doctor does not know diseases from cases or symptoms [ἀδυνατόν ἐστι προγινώσκειν τὰ τοῖς κάμνουσιν ἐσόμενα καθ' ἑκάστην νόσον]
9 *CIL*, VI, 2, 9562–617. Nos. 9563 and 9597 are the free-born foreigners
10 A. M. Duff, *Freedmen in the Early Roman Empire* (Cambridge, 1958, rpt.), 120
11 Tacitus, *Annals*, VI, 50
12 Galen, XIV, 232–3
13 Tacitus, *Annals*, XII, 61 and 67. *CIL*, VI, 8905. *IGRR*, IV, 1053, 1086 (*SIG*³, 804) 1060 (*SIG*³, 805) show Gaius Stertinius Xenophon as becoming influential at Cos. *IGRR*, IV, 1060, notes he held the Coan Eponymous Magistracy under the patronage of Claudius and apparently under Nero. *IGRR*, IV, 1086, shows alteration from *philoclaudion* to *philonerona*, after Claudius' death, and then 'friend of Nero' is also subsequently erased. E. M. Smallwood, *Documents Illustrating the Principates of Gaius, Claudius and Nero* (Cambridge, 1967), Nos. 147, 262, 289
14 Suetonius, *Augustus*, 59 and 81. Cassius Dio, LIII, 30. 3
15 *ILS*, 1842. M. McCrum and A. G. Woodhead, *Select Documents of the Principates of the Flavian Emperors* (Cambridge, 1961), 68 [no. 212]
16 *SEG*, IV, 521. E. M. Smallwood, *Documents Illustrating the Principates of Nerva, Trajan, and Hadrian* (Cambridge, 1966), 71 [no. 175]
17 H. Gummerus, *Der Ärztestand im römischen Reich nach den Inschriften* (Helsingfors, 1932 [Societas Scientiarum Fennica, Commentationes Humanarum Litterarum, III. 6]). *CIL*, VI, 5157, shows some blending of the differences between slave and free in social distinction. *CIL*, VI, 3982–7, indicate the *medici* recorded in the service of the imperial household [for Livia] were slave and free. Gummerus, 21, renders *CIL*, VI, 3986, as 'Tyrannus, slave of Livia, doctor'
18 Pliny, XXVI, 3. 4; XXIX, 8. 22. *CIL*, VI, 2594, is one of many examples of

inscriptional *medici* wealthy enough to provide their own memorials. *Cf.*
CIL, VI, 8896; XIV, 3710. *IG*, XIV., 943

19 T. Mommsen, *Römisches Staatsrecht* (Leipzig, 1887), II³. 892–6, and III, 1,
517–20. Below, 30, 57–60

20 *Codex Theodosianus*, XIII, 3. 2 [Constantine], XIII, 3. 4 [Julian], XIII, 3. 14
[Theodosius and Arcadius]. Below, 44–8. *Digest*, L, 4. 18. 30. Gummerus,
7–10

21 *SHA, Severus Alexander*, XLII, 3

22 F. Jacoby, *Die Fragmente der griechischen Historiker* (Berlin, 1929), II, 931–2
(no. 200), and *Kommentar zu Nr. 106–261* (Berlin, 1930), 626–7 (No. 200).
F. Millar, *A Study of Cassius Dio* (Oxford, 1964), 6

23 Cassius Dio, LXXX, 7. 1, and probably the same Gellius who appears in
SHA, Diadumenianus, IX, 1. The title of *archiatros* comes from the inscriptions, as well as *eques ducenarius*. *JRS*, II, 1912, 96 f., No. 25; *TAPA*, LVII
(1926), 224, No. 48; *CIL*, III, 6820; *JRS*, XIV (1924), 199, No. 35

24 B. M. Levick, *Roman Colonies in Southern Asia Minor* (Oxford, 1967), 127,
notes Gellius was a member of the Museum at Ephesus

25 *CR*, XXXIII (1919), 2, No. 1. Levick, 126

26 Ammianus Marcellinus, XVI, 6. 2–3

27 Vogt, 47–8

28 Ammianus Marcellinus, XIV, 6. 23

29 Cicero, *Ad Att.*, XV, 1a. 1. *Ad Fam.*, XIII, 20

30 Seneca, *On Benefits*, VI, 16. 1–4

31 Seneca, *On Benefits*, VI, 16. 2: 'Nihil amplius debeo.' Possibly [as Basore
translates, *LCL, Seneca: Moral Essays*, III, 397] Seneca implies 'nothing more
than his fee'. But Seneca seems to leave the sense unclear, as if to imply this
sort of doctor may not receive either gratitude or payment. This might be
particularly true of an arrogant, pompous freedman physician, such as we
read of in Galen, or of the 'theoretical physician' of whom we hear in
Polybius, XII, 25ᵉ. 4

32 Seneca, *On Benefits*, VI, 17 and 18

33 Pliny, XXVI, 7. 12–13, and XXIX, 7. 14

34 Galen, VIII, 585–7

35 Vogt, 48

36 Celsus joined practical experience with the study of books. Celsus, *Prooemium*, 28–9, 33–5, 68

37 Galen, I, 566

38 Galen, VI, 755

39 Galen, VIII, 587; VI, 755

40 Galen, VI, 552

41 Galen, V, 41; XVII, 2, 614 [Epicurean]; X, 609; XVI, 223; XIX, 59 [medi-
cine]. Galen contrasts the calm demeanour of his father with the passionate
nature of his mother, who he says was more quarrelsome than the proverbial
Xanthippe, wife of Socrates. Galen also had training in Platonic and Stoic

philosophy at an early age (14 years). P. W. Harkins, trans., *Galen On the Passions and Errors of the Soul* (Columbus, Ohio, 1963), 57. Dates for Galen's career are summarized in Singer, *Procedures*, xiii–xv

42 Galen, X, 609

43 Galen, II, 217; V, 112 [Smyrna]; II, 225; V, 119; XI, 356; XIV, 524 [Pergamon]; II, 218, 220; XVI, 136 [Alexandria]. Between his studies at Smyrna and Alexandria, Galen sat with the physician-teacher, Numesianus, at Corinth [Galen, II, 217]

44 Galen, XIII, 600; XVIII, 2, 567. Galen probably took this position to improve his knowledge of anatomy. He remarks on various matters he learned about the musculature in this period of his career. *Vid.* Galen, VI, 529; XIII, 564, 601

45 Galen, II, 215, 218

46 Galen, IV, 360

47 Galen, III, 117

48 Harkins, trans., *Galen On the Passions*, 56

49 Galen, II, 106. *Cf.* Theophrastus, *On Stones* [ed. Eichholz], V, 29

50 Galen, *On Anatomical Procedures: The Later Books*, trans. from the Arabic by W. L. H. Duckworth (Cambridge, 1962), 28 [X, 1. 34]

51 Galen, *Later Books*, 86

52 Galen, *Later Books*, 116. *Vid.* the excellent general discussion in F. J. Cole, *A History of Comparative Anatomy* (London, 1949), 42–7

53 C. P. Jones, 'A Friend of Galen', *CQ*, LXI (1967), 311–12

54 Galen, XIV, 612–29

55 Galen, II, 663–6, 673, 690, 693; 'But anyone who has seen me often doing this can be persuaded of the possibility of the experiment described, for it seems troublesome and discourages the inexperienced through the impression it makes on the mind rather than by its actual practice' [Singer, trans., *Procedures*, 219]

56 Galen, XIV, 610–29

57 Galen, II, 642–5. Singer, trans., 197–8

58 Galen, VII, 478; XIV, 201, 206, 216; XIX, 18. *Vid.* T. W. Africa, 'The Opium Addiction of Marcus Aurelius', *JHI*, XXII (1961), 97–102

59 Galen, V, 527 and 544 contrasted with XVII, 2, 135–43

60 J. S. Kieffer, trans., *Galen's Institutio Logica* (Baltimore, 1964), 1–18 [introd.]

61 De Lacy O'Leary, *How Greek Science Passed to the Arabs* (London, 1949), 34–5; E. G. Browne, *Arabian Medicine* (Cambridge, 1962), 21, 25–8, 55, 63; and N. Rescher, *Galen and the Syllogism* (Pittsburgh, 1966)

62 S. Sambursky, *The Physical World of Late Antiquity* (London, 1962), 41

63 Sambursky, 40

64 Sambursky, 39

65 Galen, I, 560

66 Galen, I, 566

67 Galen, I, 561

68 May, *Parts*, 45. Galen's physiological theories have received much attention. O. Temkin, 'On Galen's Pneumatology', *Gesnerus*, VIII (1951), 180–9. N. Mani, *Die historische Grundlagen der Leberforschung* (Basel/Stuttgart, 1965), I, 65–72. L. G. Wilson, 'Erasistratus, Galen, and the *Pneuma*,' *BHM*, XXXIII (1959), 293–314, and 'The Problem of the Discovery of the Pulmonary Circulation', *JHM*, XVII (1962), 229–44. R. E. Siegel, *Galen's System of Physiology and Medicine* (Basel/New York, 1968). V. A. Triolo, 'An Interpretive Analysis of Galenic Renal Physiology', *Clio Medica*, I (1966), 113–28

69 Galen, II, 4–5, 7–9, 167–8 (Brock, 8–9, 12–15, 258–61)

70 Galen, IV, 767–822, among many examples. *Vid.* May, *Parts*, 44–6

71 Galen, IV, 688–702

72 The retiform plexus is found in ungulates but not in man. In man, the area is occupied by the Circle of Willis. *Cf.* Galen, *Usefulness of Parts*, IX, 4 (May, 430–4)

73 Galen, *Usefulness of Parts*, VI, 17 (May, 324)

74 Galen, *Usefulness of Parts*, VIII, 6 (May, 399). Galen, V, 600–17 (May, 399ff, note 42)

75 Galen, X, 839–40

76 May, *Parts*, 49, with ref. to Galen, II, 1–214 (Brock)

77 Galen, II, 9–10 (Brock, 16–17)

78 Galen, IX, 935

79 Galen, IX, 935

80 Galen, XII, 207

81 Galen, IX, 910–11

82 Galen, IX, 912

83 Galen, IX, 913. *Cf.* Pseudo-Galen, *Prognostica de decubitu ex mathematica scientia* (Kühn, XIX, 529–73), which is a detailed medico-astrological treatise. *CIG*, 5821, tells us that one Decius Servillius Apollonius, a physician, died at the age of ninety-three, having predicted his own death through astrology

84 Suetonius, *Augustus*, 45. *BGU*, 1074. *London Papyrus*, III, 1178. Herzog, 975–6. *SHA*, *Severus Alexander*, XLIV, 4

85 Galen, XIV, 90–209

86 *SHA*, *Hadrian*, XXIII, 16. Aelius Verus is apparently killed by an overdose of drugs

87 *Digest*, L, 4. 18. 30. *Cf. Digest*, XXVII, 1. 6. 8–12 [the physician-teacher has to perform in his home town], Julian, *Orations*, VII, 207 D, and *Digest*, XXXVIII, 1. 25–7 [the relation between the aristocrat and his physician]

88 Varro, *De lingua Latina*, VII, 4

89 Varro, *De lingua Latina*, V, 93

90 Varro, *De lingua Latina*, V, 8

91 Varro, *De lingua Latina*, X, 46

92 Cicero, *On the Orator*, I, 62; *On Duties*, I, 150–1. Seneca, *Questions Naturelles* [ed. Otramare (Budé)], II, 38. 4. *Digest*, L, 9. 4. 2. Macrobius, *Saturnalia*,

VII, 4. 1–33 and VII, 15. 15
93 Pliny, XXVI, 3. 4
94 Pliny, XXIX, 8. 22
95 Galen, XIV, 647
96 Galen, VIII, 224
97 Galen, XIII, 597
98 R. Walzer, trans., from the Arabic, *Galen On Medical Experience* (Oxford, 1944), 142

CHAPTER IX

1 Marrou, 302. Super-specialization has not, however, hindered the European physician's role in the twentieth century. J. Mitchener, *Iberia* (New York, 1968), 571–3, comments on the doctor's prestige in modern Spain. The physician is the most durable of the 'liberals' in Spain because of his 'prepared position' which he can fall back upon in case his liberal tendencies run into official opposition. The same seems to be true of Italy and Greece in the twentieth century. Doctors seem to be the most widely read, own the most books, exhibit the broadest learning, and, in the smaller towns, have the best houses
2 L. Edelstein, 'Recent Trends in the Interpretation of Ancient Science', *JHI*, XIII (1952), 573–604, which rejects emphasis upon slavery, and is particularly a critique of B. Farrington, *Head and Hand in Ancient Greece* (London, 1947), chs. I and II. Marrou, 302
3 Marrou, 303
4 For example, Galen, I, 53–63, among many
5 Jaeger, *Paideia*, III, 3
6 Galen, III, 74 and 364
7 Galen, II, 475, 681, 696; IV, 685; V, 289. Oribasius, III, 236
8 I. E. Drabkin, 'On Medical Education in Greece and Rome', *BHM*, XV (1944), 333–51 [334]
9 For example his total or partial sectioning of the spinal column, or of various nerves, or of the experiments in which he sliced the brain in layers etc. [in pigs]. Galen, II, 677, 682, 692, 697; V, 645
10 Galen, III, 644
11 Galen, IV, 487
12 Marrou, 303
13 Plato, *Laws*, IV, 720A–E. *Cf.* P. Lain-Entralgo, 'Die ärztliche Hilfe im Werk Platons', *AGM*, XLVI (1962), 193–210
14 Aristotle, *De sensu*, 436a
15 Aristotle, *Politics*, III, 1282a. 11: the craftsman, or ordinary practitioner (δημιουργός), the specialist or scientist-physician (ἀρχιτεκτονικός), and the man who has studied the art (ὁ πεπαιδευμένος περὶ τὴν τέχνην)

16 *Ibid.* The translation is that of E. Barker. *The Politics of Aristotle* (Oxford, 1962), 125
17 Plato, *Protagoras*, 313 D. Similar to *Gorgias*, 450 A and 517 E
18 Plato, *Gorgias*, 464 B
19 Plato, *Sophist*, 226 E–227 A
20 Plato, *Sophist*, 228D–229A. Περὶ μὲν αἶσχος γυμναστική, περὶ δὲ νόσον ἰατρική
21 Plato, *Republic*, III, 406A–B. Plato goes on to condemn the 'modern' tendency of medical 'valetudinarianism'
22 C. A. Forbes, 'Accidents and Fatalities in Greek Athletics', in *Classical Studies in Honor of W. A. Oldfather* (Urbana, Illinois, 1943), 50–9, and R. S. Robinson, *Sources for the History of Greek Athletics* (Cincinnati, 1955), 176, 217–18
23 Jaeger, *Paideia*, III, 4. Plutarch, *The Education of Children*, 7E, echoes Plato
24 Celsus, *Prooemium*, 7
25 *Ibid.*, 9
26 *Ibid.*, 29–30
27 *Ibid.*, 39
28 *Ibid.*, 48
29 *Ibid.*, 52–3. Cf. 70
30 *Ibid.*, 73
31 Oribasius, III, 164 (Vol. IV, 139, ed. Raeder), quoting Athenaeus
32 Drabkin, 'Medical Education', 334
33 Galen, XIX, 50
34 From the writings of Archibus (1st century AD), as given in H. Schöne, *Berliner Klass. Texte*, III (1905), 24. English translation from Drabkin, 'Medical Education', 335
35 Galen, XIV, 674–797 (678–83 on sects)
36 Galen, XIX, 21. Lucian, *Remarks to an Illiterate Book-Fancier*, 29
37 Plautus, *Amphitruo*, IV, 4
38 Galen, XVIII, 2. 678
39 Galen, XVIII, 2, 629–925
40 Celsus, *Prooemium*, 65. Columella, XI, 1; XII, 3. Tacitus, *Dialogue on Oratory*, 21. The Talmud defines clearly apprenticeships for physicians. E. M. Heichelheim, 'Roman Syria', in T. Frank, ed., *Economic Survey of Ancient Rome* (Baltimore, 1938), IV, 199
41 Martial, V. 9. Philostratus, *Apollonius of Tyana*, VIII, 7. 14
42 Galen, I, 83; X, 5 and 19
43 Pliny, XXIX, 8. 17–18
44 Galen, XIX, 9
45 Lucian, *Disowned Son*, 3–4, 13–16, 23–4, 29–31. Lucian, *Hippias*, 1, remarks that the public reacted more kindly to doctors with practical training than to those who made speeches on the healing art
46 Lucian, *Disowned Son*, 4

47 Galen, II, 220 (Singer, *Procedures*, 3). The tradition of medical illustrations from antiquity is probably preserved in extant medieval manuscripts. L. MacKinney, *Medical Illustrations in Medieval Manuscripts* (Berkeley, 1965), e.g. 16 (pl. 11), 28 (pl. 20), 70 (pl. 69). *Cf.* E. Holländer, *Die Medizin in der classischen Malerei* (Berlin, 1913); B. F. Horine, 'An Epitome of Ancient Pulse Lore', *BHM*, X (1941), 216–35; and H. Schöne, ed., *Apollonius von Kitium: illustrierter Kommentar zu der hippokratischen Schrift* (Leipzig, 1896)

48 Galen, II, 631–4 (Singer, 191–3)

49 Galen, II, 222 (Singer, 3). Singer, 240 (note 22), notes that the Rhesus monkey (*Macaca mulatta*) was the usual choice

50 Galen, II, 633 (Singer, 193)

51 Galen, II, 385–6 (Singer, 77)

52 Rufus, 34

53 Galen, II, 218–21 (Singer, 2–3)

54 Aulus Gellius, XVIII, 10

55 Rufus, 219–32

56 Aretaeus, *On Acute Diseases*, II, 3. Galen, XVIII, 2, 649

57 Lucretius, VI, 5. 112–14. Celsus, III, 25. Aretaeus, *On Chronic Diseases*, II, 13, [leprosy]. Galen, XVII, 1, 351 [diarrhoea]. Galen, XVII, 2, 742 [jaundice]. Celsus, III, 22. Aretaeus, *On Chronic Diseases*, I, 8 [tuberculosis]. The symptoms of tuberculosis are clear in Pliny the Younger, *Letters*, VII, 19. *Vid.* E. F. Lear, 'A Case of Tuberculosis in the Roman Aristocracy at the Beginning of the Second Century', *JHM*, XIV (1959), 86–8

58 Aretaeus, *On Acute Diseases*, I, 9

59 Galen, VIII, 73

60 Aretaeus, *On Chronic Diseases*, I, 7

61 Dioscorides, I, 2. Bassus commanded the Roman army at the successful siege of Machaerus in Judaea (AD 71). Flavius Josephus, *Jewish War*, VII, 6

62 Galen, XI, 858, 443, 794

63 Galen, XIV, 30

64 Galen, XI, 797

65 Pliny, XXV, 8, 27

66 Galen, XIII, 570. For Roman botany, M. Wellmann, 'Sextus Niger, eine Quellenuntersuchung zu Dioscorides', *Hermes*, XXIV (1889), 530–69 [noting that Pliny and Dioscorides both use Sextus Niger], and J. Stannard, 'Pliny and Roman Botany', *Isis*, LVI (1965), 420–5 [argues for Pliny's ability in botany], provide a glance at the problems in this area

67 Pliny, XXXIV, 25. 108

68 Galen, XII, 216; XIV, 7ff

69 Galen, XII, 216

70 Galen, XIV, 7

71 Galen, XIII, 571

72 Galen, XIV, 83ff. G. Watson, *Theriac and Mithridatium* (London, 1966), 64–93

73 O. Temkin, 'Studies in Late Alexandrian Medicine I', *BHM*, III (1935), 405–30 [423–4]

74 Ammianus Marcellinus, XXII, 16. 18. *Vid.* J. Scarborough, 'Ammianus Marcellinus XXII, 16. 18: Alexandria's Medical Reputation in the Fourth Century', *Clio Medica* IV (1969) [forthcoming]

75 Galen, II, 215–18 (Singer, 1–2): *Anatomical Procedures.* Galen, II, 227–9 (Singer, 5–6): *Muscles.* Galen, II, 220, 223–7, 732–78 (Singer's translation in *PRS*, XLV (1952), 25–34): *Bones*

76 Galen, II, 227–8. Singer translates roughly the same with different phrasing (Singer, 6)

77 Galen, VI, 164–5

78 Soranus, *Gynecology*, I, 1. 1 (Temkin, 4)

79 Drabkin, 'Medical Education', 349

80 *CIL*, VI, 9566, 29805; IX, 1618. J. Keil, 'Ärzteininschriften aus Ephesos', *Jahresheft d. Österreichischen Arch. Inst.*, VIII (1905), 128–38, notes the parallel in the Greek half of the Roman world and the preceding tradition

81 Herzog, 972, 1001. Below, 30 *Cf.* Julian, *Letters*, 31

82 *Codex Theodosianus*, XIII, 3. 5 and 3. 8. 2

83 *SHA, Alexander Severus*, 44

84 *Codex Theodosianus*, XIII, 3. 1. 2, and 3. 3

85 T. R. S. Broughton, 'Roman Asia Minor', in T. Frank, ed., *Economic Survey of Ancient Rome* (Baltimore, 1938), IV, 806

86 *IGRR*, IV, 446

87 Broughton, 'Roman Asia', 806–7

88 *Digest*, XXVII, 1, 6, 2–4

89 Broughton, 'Roman Asia', 851, with refs. The important inscription speaking of associations of physicians reads τὸ συνέδριον, οἱ ἐν 'Εφέσῳ ἀπὸ τοῦ Μουσείου ἰατροί. *Cf.* Keil's study (cited in note 80 above)

CHAPTER X

1 S. K. de Waard, 'Les idées psychiatriques des juristes romains', *PIC*² (Paris, 1921), 175–7

2 F. Zibordi, 'La tutelle de l'enfant dans l'empire grec-égyptien et dans l'empire romain', *PIC*² (Paris, 1921), 526–9. Reinforced by *BGU*, I, 297; IV, 1106–12, 1153, 1158

3 *SEHRE*, I, 182, 358–9 [with plate LXX, no. 1]. *CAH*, XI, 210–11, 887 [bibliography on the problems of the *alimenta*]

4 *SEHRE*, I, 364 [plate LXXI] shows an *aureus* of Trajan and the symbolic distribution of money to needy children

5 A. C. Lloyd in review of E. R. Dodds, *Pagan and Christian in an Age of Anxiety* (Cambridge, 1965), in *JRS*, LVI (1966), 254, suggests this idea, using the English context

6 Galen, *On Medical Experience*, XIX (Walzer, trans., 121)
7 Galen, *On Medical Experience*, XVIII–XX
8 D. Morris, *The Naked Ape* (New York, 1967), 208
9 W. R. Miles, 'Chimpanzee Behaviour: Removal of a Foreign Body from a Companion's Eye', *Proceedings of the National Academy of Sciences*, XLIX (1963), 235–7, and J. van Hooff, 'Facial Expression in Higher Primates', *Symposia of the Zoological Society of London*, VIII (1962), 97–125
10 Morris, 209
11 Morris, 209
12 Morris, 209–10
13 Plutarch, *Superstition*, 7 (168 C)
14 Plutarch, *Letter to Apollonius*, 12 (107 F). *Cf.* 10 (106 D) where he quotes Aeschylus
15 Plutarch, *On Listening to Lectures*, 16 (46 E)
16 Plutarch, *How to Tell a Flatterer from a Friend*, 20 (61 D)
17 Plutarch, *Flatterer*, 22 (63 D)
18 Plutarch, *Advice to Bride and Groom*, 22 (141 B)
19 Plutarch, *How to Profit by One's Enemies*, 6 (89 C)
20 Propertius, II, 1. 57–70, begins: Omnes humanos sanat medicina dolores/ solus amor morbi non amat artificem. Then we read of Machaon, Chiron, the 'Epidauran' god, and so on
21 Plutarch, *Flatterer*, 36 (73 D)
22 Plutarch, *How to Study Poetry*, 8 (26 C)
23 Plutarch, *Dinner of the Seven Wise Men*, 14 (158 A–B). *Cf.* Hesiod, *Works and Days*, 405–821 (daily course), 368–9 (wine), 595, 737–41 (water), 736–41, 753 (bathing), 373–5, 699–705 (women), 735–6, 812 (sexual relations), and 750–2 (infants)
24 Plutarch, *Introduction to Health*, 26 (136 E–F)
25 Plutarch, *Introduction to Health*, 26 (137 A)
26 Plutarch, *How a Man May Become Aware of his Progress in Virtue*, 11 (81 F–82 A)
27 Plutarch, *Letter to Apollonius*, 22 (112 F). *Cf.* Plato, *Republic*, X, 6 C–E (604 C–E), Demosthenes, IV, 40 (51), Sophocles, *Ajax*, 582, and Ovid, *Metamorphoses*, I, 190
28 Plutarch, *Flatterer*, 37 (74 D)
29 Plutarch, *Letter to Apollonius*, 2 (102 A). *Cf.* Cicero, *Tusculan Disputations*, IV, 29. 63, and Pliny, *Letters*, V, 16
30 Plutarch, *Flatterer*, 11 (54 E)
31 Plutarch, *Flatterer*, 11 (55 A–B). *Cf.* Pliny, XXI, 7. 44 and XXI, 20. 145 (polium)
32 Plutarch, *Flatterer*, 17 (60 B)
33 Plutarch, *Flatterer*, 27 (67 F)
34 Plutarch, *Introduction to Health*, 20 (133 C)
35 Plutarch, *Advice to Bride and Groom*, 20 (140 E)

36 Plutarch, *Dinner of the Seven Wise Men*, 10 (154 C). Plutarch says one Cleodorus invented this method (fl. under Solon)

37 Plutarch, *Progress in Virtue*, 8 (80 A)

38 Plutarch, *Introduction to Health*, 11 (128 A)

39 Aretaeus of Cappadocia, *Acute Diseases*, I, 6. Text F. Adams, *The Extant Works of Aretaeus, the Cappadocian* (London, 1856), 9–10

40 Adams, trans., 293

41 Adams, trans., 293–4

42 Adams, trans., 421

43 Galen, IX, 217–20 (boasts he has never made a mistake in diagnosis, prognosis, or judgement in his medical practice)

44 Aretaeus, *Acute Diseases* (Therapeutics), II, 9. Celsus, VII, 26

45 Celsus, *Prooemium*, 52–3

46 Celsus, *Prooemium*, 54

47 Celsus, *Prooemium*, 51–2: Cum igitur talis res incidit, medicus aliquid oportet inveniat, quod non utique fortasse sed saepius tamen etiam respondeat

48 Galen, II, 128: ... ἥτις ἂν ἐν τῷ σώματι διάθεσις βλάπτῃ τὴν ἐνέργειαν μὴ κατά τι συμβεβηκὸς ἀλλὰ πρῶτός τε καὶ καθ' ἑαυτήν, αὕτη τὸ νόσημά ἐστιν αὐτό. Πῶς οὖν ἔτι διαγνωστικός τε καὶ ἰατρικὸς ἔσται τῶν νοσημάτων ἀγνοῶν ὅλως αὐτὰ τίνα τ' ἐστὶ καὶ πόσα καὶ ποῖα;

49 B. Farrington, *Greek Science* (Baltimore, 1961), 304–5

50 E.g. Galen, XVII, 2, 135–43

51 Britain: *CIL*, VII, 431 (Lancaster), *CIL*, VII, 164 (Chester). Phoenicia: Strabo, XVI, 2. 22 (Asclepion between Berytus and Sidon). Black Sea: Strabo, II, 2. 16 (Panticapaion). Egypt: Aelian, *On Animals*, XVI, 39 (Alexandria), Ammianus Marcellinus, XXII, 14. 7 and Tacitus, *Histories*, IV, 84 (Memphis), *CIG*, 4894 (Philis). Africa: *CIL*, VIII, 2, 9320 (Mauretania), *CIL*, VIII, 1, 2579–90 and 2624 (Lambaesis), Strabo, XVII, 3. 14 (Carthage), Pausanias, II, 26. 9, *CIG*, 5131, and Tacitus, *Annals*, XIV, 18 (Cyrene). Spain: Polybius, X, 10. 8 (New Carthage), *CIL*, II, 21 (Merobriga), *CIL*, II, 3819 (Saguntum), and CIL, II, 3725–6 (Valentia). The heaviest concentration of sanctuaries was in Greece and Asia Minor, and the evidence, both literary and epigraphical, is overwhelming. E.g. Pausanias, X, 4. 4 and 32. 12 (Phocis); Cicero, *On the Nature of the Gods*, III, 22. 56 and Pausanias, IX, 39. 4 (Boeotia); Xenophon, *Memorabilia*, III, 13. 3 and Pausanias, I, 21. 4 (Athens' Acropolis); Pausanias, I, 40. 6 (Megara); Pausanias, II, 2. 3 and II, 4. 5 (Corinth); Pausanias, II, 10. 2 and IV, 14. 8 (Sicyon); Pausanias, II, 23. 4 (Argos); Strabo, VIII, 16. 15, and Cicero, *On the Nature of the Gods*, IV, 34. 83 (Epidaurus. This was the temple robbed by Sulla: Diodorus Siculus, XXXVIII, 7); Pausanias, VIII, 28. 1 (Gortys in Arcadia); Pausanias, VIII, 47. 1 and 54. 5 (Tegea); Strabo, VIII, 3. 4 (Cyllene in Elis; Pausanias, IV, 31. 10 (Messene); *CIG*, 1392 (Gythium); Pausanias, III, 26. 4 (Leuctra); Pausanias, III, 14. 2 and 15. 10 (Sparta); *CIG*, 2046 (Hadrianopolis in Thrace); *CIG*,

3158–9, 3170, and Pausanias, II, 26. 9 (Smyrna); Strabo, XIV, 2. 20 and Tacitus, *Annals*, IV, 14 (Cos); *CIG*, 364lb (Lampsacus); *CIG*, 2038 (Pera in Macedonia); *CIG*, 3582 (Troy); Pausanias, II, 26. 8; Tacitus, *Annals*, III, 63; *CIG*, 3538; Polybius, XXXII, 8. 15, and Galen, *passim*. (Pergamon); *CIG*, 4315n (Rhodiopolis in Lycia); Arrian, *Anabasis of Alexander*, II, 5. 8 and Quintus Curtius, III, 7. 3 (Soli in Cilicia); *CIL*, III, 1, 242 and *CIG*, 3428 (Ancyra in Galatia). Most of the important evidence for geographic distribution of the cult is collected in Edelstein, *Asclepius*, I, 370–452 (*CIL*, VII, 431, 164, and Strabo, II, 2. 16, are not included)

52 Galen, XIV, 674 (Apollo, the father of Asclepius). Ovid, *Metamorphoses*, II, 630 (Asclepius educated by Chiron). Edelstein, *Asclepius*, I, 1–178

53 Pliny, II, 1–5; XXII, 1 and 7. 14–17; XXV, 1–6; XXXVII. 1

54 *IG*, IV, 121–4, 417, 424–5, 438

55 Aelius Aristides, *Sacred Tales*, V (Keil, *Oratio*, 51, 57–67)

56 A. Panayotatou, 'Terres cuites d'Égypte de l'époque Gréco-Romain, et maladies', *PIC*[6] (Amsterdam, 1927), 41–7. K. Sudhoff, *Ärztliches aus griechischen Papyrus-Urkunden* (Leipzig, 1909), 200

57 Servius, *Commentarii in Virgilium* (ed. Lion), XI, 785. *CIL*, I, 1. 231

58 Pausanias, II, 26. 3–5

59 Vitruvius, I, 2. 7. Plutarch, *Roman Questions*, 94 (286 D)

60 Servius, *Commentarii*, X, 316 (infants born 'Caesarian' were sacred to Apollo)

61 Horace, *Epistulae*, I, 34–41. Trans. S. P. Bovie, *Satires and Epistles of Horace* (Chicago, 1959), 166

62 Galen, XIV, 631; XVIII, 2, 40

63 *Digest*, L, 13. 1. 3. *Cf.* Josephus, *Jewish Antiquities*, VIII, 2. 5, and Matthew, XII, 27

64 Dioscorides, IV, 151

65 Libanius, *Orations*, I, 143, 244 (ed. and trans. A. F. Norman, *Libanius' Autobiography* (Oxford, 1965), 83, 244). Some problems of magic and its strong appeal are surveyed in A. A. Barb, 'The Survival of Magic Arts', in A. Momigliano, ed., *The Conflict Between Paganism and Christianity in the Fourth Century* (Oxford, 1964), 100–25

66 L. Thorndike, *History of Magic and Experimental Science* (New York, 1923), I, 268–86. Cicero, *On Divination*, II, 59. 122–3, shows some of the Roman intellectual's attitude toward medical instruction given in dreams. Cicero uses the lack of a parallel for Neptune giving instruction for seafaring, nor do the Muses instruct in reading or writing in dreams. Thus *medicina* cannot result from dreams.

67 Hopkins, 125

68 E. R. Dodds, *The Greeks and the Irrational* (Berkeley, 1963)

APPENDIX II

1 In participating in a dig at the Jordanian site of Machaerus (summer, 1968), I occasionally ran across coins which would lead one to believe the fortress was destroyed several decades before the Romans actually took it. If we did not have Flavius Josephus' more-or-less eyewitness account of the Jewish surrender (AD 71), we might be completely at the mercy of these scattered coins

2 *Cf.* Charles Singer's remarks in his translation of *Galen On Anatomical Procedures* (Oxford, 1956), xx–xxi

3 The trend seems to be changing. *Cf.* R. J. Durling, 'Lectiones Galenicae', *CP*, LXIII (1968), 56–7

4 According to a letter received from the Licht Foundation in New Haven, Connecticut, further translations of Galen by R. M. Green (as listed in Sarton, *Galen of Pergamon*, 106) remain in manuscript form, but have not yet been scheduled for publication

5 Athenaeus, I, 1e–f. Galen is described as 'having published more books on philosophy and medicine than all those before him', and he is contrasted with Daphnus of Ephesus who is 'of pure character and skilled in the art'

SOURCES OF ILLUSTRATIONS

The author and publishers are grateful to the many official bodies and individuals listed below who have supplied illustrations.

Mansell-Alinari, 1, 13, 14, 18, 23, 31, 32, 36, 40, 43, 47, 48; Trustees of the British Museum, 2, 3, 11, 30, 33, 34, 37, 38, 39, 41, 42, 44, 45, 46; R. Bessier, Friburg, 4; Vatican Museums, 5; Piacenza Museum, 6; Department of the History of Medicine, Kansas University Medical Center, 7; City of Liverpool Museums, 8; Professor Pericle di Pietro, 9, 10; Foteteca Unione, 12, 24, 25, 26, 28, 29, 35; J. Bottin, Paris, 15; Casanatese Library, Rome, 16 (ms. 1382, fol. 25); Bologna University, 17 (ms. 3652, fol. 51); German Archaeological Institute, Rome, 19, 49; Rhein. Landesmuseum, Bonn, 20, 21; American Academy in Rome, 22; V. E. Nash-Williams, 27

Figures 1, 15, and 17 were drawn by T. Hardaker; 10, 11, 12 and 16 by Miss G. Jones, and 3, 7, 8 and 9 by M. Ricketts. Figures 4 and 5 are reproduced by kind permission of the Society for the Promotion of Roman Studies.

The author particularly wishes to express his thanks and appreciation to Professor Pericle di Pietro for providing plates 9 and 10 and for his comment upon them, and also to Mr D. Bailey of the Department of Greek and Roman Antiquities, British Museum, for his help with plate 11 and his rewarding discussion of this lamp.

P

BIBLIOGRAPHY

SOURCES AND EDITIONS

AETIUS   Olivieri, A., ed., *Aetii Amideni Libri medicinales V–VIII*. Berlin, 1950
Ricci, J. V., trans., *Aetios of Amida*. Philadelphia, 1950

ANONYMUS LONDINENSIS   Jones, W. H. S., ed., *The Medical Writings of Anonymus Londinensis*. Cambridge, 1947

ANTONIUS MUSA   Howald, E., ed., *De herba vettonica liber*. Leipzig, 1927

ARETAEUS OF CAPPADOCIA   Adams, F., ed. and trans., *The Extant Works of Aretaeus the Cappadocian*. London, 1856
Hude, C., ed., *Aretaeus*. Berlin, 1958
Kühn, C. G., ed. (Aretaeus) *Opera*. Leipzig, 1828

CAELIUS AURELIANUS   Drabkin, I. E., ed. and trans., *Caelius Aurelianus on Acute Diseases and on Chronic Diseases*. Chicago, 1950

CELSUS   Spencer, W. G., ed., and trans., *Celsus De medicina*. *LCL*. 3 vols.

DIOSCORIDES   Goodyer, J., trans., and Gunther, R. T., ed., *Dioscorides Greek Herbal*. New York, 1959 (rpt)
Wellmann, M., ed., *Pedanii Dioscuridis de materia medica*. 3 vols. Berlin, 1958 (rpt)

ERASISTRATUS   Dobson, J. F., 'Erasistratus,' *PRS*, XX (1927), 825–32

GALEN   Brock, A. J., ed., and trans., *Galen on the Natural Faculties*. *LCL*
Duckworth, W. L. H., trans. from the Arabic, *Galen on Anatomical Procedures. The Later Books*. Cambridge, 1962
Harkins, P. W., trans., *Galen on the Passions and Errors of the Soul*. Columbus, Ohio, 1963
Kieffer, J. S., trans., *Galen's Institutio Logica*. Baltimore, 1964
Kühn, C. G., ed., *Galenus Opera Omnia*. 20 vols in 22. Hildesheim, 1964–5 (rpt)
May, M. T., trans., *Galen on the Usefulness of the Parts of the Body*. 2 vols. Ithaca, New York, 1968
Singer, C., trans., *Galen on Anatomical Procedures*. Oxford, 1956

HERODOTUS   Wellmann, M., 'Herodots Werk', *Hermes*, XL (1905), 580–604

HEROPHILUS   Dobson, J. F., 'Herophilus of Alexandria', *PRS*, XVIII (1925), 19–32

HIPPOCRATES   Jones, W. H. S., and Withington, E. T., eds., and transls., *Hippocrates*. 4 vols. *LCL*
Littré, E., ed. and French trans., *Hippocrates Œuvres complètes*. 10 vols. Paris, 1839–61

ORIBASIUS   Bussemaker, U. C., and Daremberg, C., eds. and French transls., *Oribasius Œuvres*. 6 vols. Paris, 1851–76
Raeder, I., ed., *Oribasii collectionum medicarum reliquiae*. 5 vols. Amsterdam, 1964 (rpt)

PAUL   Adams, F., trans., *The Seven Books of Paulus Aegineta*. 3 vols. London, 1844–7

PLINY   Jones, W. H. S., and Eichholz, D. E., eds. and transls., *Pliny Natural History*. 10 vols. *LCL*

RUFUS OF EPHESUS   Daremberg, C., and Ruelle, C. E., eds. and French transls., (Rufus of Ephesus) *Œuvres*. Amsterdam, 1963 (rpt)

SCRIBONIUS LARGUS   Helmreich, G., ed. (Scribonius Largus) *Compositiones*. Leipzig, 1887

(Quintus) SERENUS SAMMONICUS   Pépin, R., ed., and French trans. (Serenus Sammonicus) *Liber medicinalis*. Paris, 1950
Vollmer, F., ed. (Serenus Sammonicus) *Liber medicinalis*. Leipzig, 1916

SORANUS   Temkin, O., trans., *Soranus' Gynecology*. Baltimore, 1956

THEODORUS PRISCIANUS   Meyer, T., *Theodorus Priscianus und die römische Medizin*. Jena, 1909. German trans. of *Euphoriston*
Rose, V., ed., *Theodorus Priscianus Euphoriston libri III*. Leipzig, 1894

THEOPHILUS and LEO   Ermerins, F. Z., ed., *Anecdota medica Graeca*. Amsterdam, 1963 (rpt). Byzantine medicine. Contains Theophilus, *De pulsibus*, Leo, *Philosophi conspectus medicinae*, the uncertain *E libro de medicina ad Constantinum Pognatum imperatorem*, and the *Hippocratis epistola ad Ptolemaeum regem de hominis fabrica*.

SOURCE BOOKS AND SOURCE COLLECTIONS

Brock, A. J., *Greek Medicine*. London, 1929
Clendening, L. G., ed., *Source Book of Medical History*. New York, 1960 (rpt)
Cohen, M. R., and Drabkin, I. E., *A Source Book in Greek Science*. Harvard, 1958
Müri, W., *Der Arzt im Altertum*. Munich, 1962

BIBLIOGRAPHICAL GUIDES

Artelt, W., *Einführung in die Medizinhistorik*. Stuttgart, 1949
Drabkin, M., 'A Select Bibliography of Greek and Roman Medicine', *BHM*, XI (1942), 399–408
Sarton, G., *Introduction to the History of Science*. Vol. I. Washington, 1927
Wellcome Institute, *Current Work in the History of Medicine. International Bibliography*. Issued quarterly (Euston Road, London, N.W. 1)

SUPPLEMENTARY BIBLIOGRAPHY

The following were consulted but are not cited in the notes

GENERAL HISTORIES

Diepgen, P., *Geschichte der Medizin*. 2 vols in 3. Berlin, 1949–55
Garrison, F., *An Introduction to the History of Medicine*. 4th ed. London, 1929
Laignel-Lavastine, M. (ed.), *Histoire général de la médecine, de la pharmacie, de l'art dentaire*. 3 vols. Paris, 1936–49
Major, R. H., *A History of Medicine*. 2 vols. Springfield, Illinois, 1954
Meyer-Steineg, T., and Sudhoff, K., *Illustrierte Geschichte der Medizin*. 5th ed. (R. Herrlinger and F. Kudlien). Stuttgart, 1965

Pazzini, A., *Storia della medicina*. 2 vols. Milan, 1947
Singer, C., *A Short History of Anatomy and Physiology from the Greeks to Harvey*. New York, 1957 (rpt)

THE BACKGROUND OF CLASSICAL SCIENCE

Charlesworth, M. P., *Trade-Routes and Commerce of the Roman Empire*. Cambridge, 1924
Clagett, M., *Greek Science in Antiquity*. New York, 1963
Farrington, B., *Science and Politics in the Ancient World*. London, 1965
Kranzberg, M., and Pursell, C. W. Jr., *Technology in Western Civilization*. Vol. I. Oxford, 1967
Miller, J. I., *The Spice Trade of the Roman Empire*. Oxford, 1969
Moritz, L. A., *Grain-Mills and Flour in Classical Antiquity*. Oxford, 1958
Neugebauer, O., *The Exact Sciences in Antiquity*. New York, 1962 (rpt)
Sambursky, S., *The Physical World of the Greeks*. New York, 1962 (rpt)
Singer, C., *From Magic to Science*. New York, 1958
White, K. D., *Agricultural Implements of the Roman World*. Cambridge, 1967
White, Lynn, *Medieval Technology and Social Change*. Oxford, 1962

SPECIAL STUDIES

Allbutt, T. C., *Greek Medicine in Rome*. London, 1921
Amacher, M. P., 'Galen's Experiment on the Arterial Pulse and the Experiment Repeated', *AGM*, XLVIII (1964), 177–80
Baader, G., 'Ueberlieferungsprobleme des A. Cornelius Celsus', *Forschungen und Fortschritte*, XXXIV (1960), 215–18
Blanchard, R., *Épigraphie médicale*. 2 vols. Paris, 1909–15
Boswinkel, E., 'La médecine et les médecins dans les papyrus Grecs', *Eos*, XLVIII (1956), 181–90
Bullock, F., 'Mulomedicina Chironis', *PIC³*, 304–5
Carstens, H. R., 'The History of Hospitals with Special Reference to some of the World's Oldest Institutions', *Annals of Internal Medicine*, X, (1937), 670–82
Collinge, N. E., 'Medical Terms and Clinical Attitudes in the Tragedians', *Bulletin of the Institute of Classical Studies of the University of London*, IX (1962), 43–55
Didsbury, G., 'Considérations sur la migraine d'après Arétée de Cappadoce', *Bulletin de la Société Française d'Histoire de la Médecine*, XXX (1936), 260–7
Deichgräber, K., 'Ausgewähltes aus der medizinischen Literatur der Antike', *Philologus*, CI (1957), 135–47
Drabkin, I. E., 'Soranus and his System of Medicine', *BHM*, XXV (1951), 503–18
    'Remarks on Ancient Psychotherapy,' *Isis*, XLVI (1955), 223–34
Eichholz, D. E., 'Galen and his Environment', *GR*, XX (1951), 60–71
Esser, A., *Das Antlitz der Blindheit in der Antike*. Leiden, 1961
Evans, E. C., 'Galen the Physician as Physiognomist', *TAPA* (1945), 287–98
Franke, F., *Über die Augenheilkunde des Celsus*. Berlin, 1898
Garrison, F. H., *Notes on the History of Military Medicine*. Washington, 1922

Gazza, V., 'Prescrizioni mediche nei papiri del'Egitto Greco-Romano', *Aegyptus*, XXXV (1955), 86–110

Heinecke, W., *Zahnärztliches in den Werken des Oreibasios*. Leipzig, 1922

Iftner, H., *Die Zahnheilkunde bei Aulus Cornelius Celsus*. Würzburg, 1925

Jones, W. H. S., *Malaria and Greek History*. Manchester, 1909

Jüthner, J., *Körperkultur im Altertum*. Jena, 1928

Kollesch, J., 'Galen und seine ärtzlichen Kollegen', *Das Altertum*, XI (1965), 47–53

Kudlien, F., 'Probleme um Diokles von Karystos', *AGM*, XLVII (1963), 456–64
'The Third Century A.D.—A Blank Spot in the History of Medicine?' in *Medicine, Science, and Culture. Historical Essays in Honor of Owsei Temkin*, ed. L. G. Stevenson and R. P. Multhauf (Baltimore, 1968), 25–34
Untersuchungen zu Aretaios von Kappadokien. Wiesbaden, 1964

Mani, N., 'Die Nachtblindheit und ihre Behandlung in der griechisch-römischen Medizin', *Gesnerus*, X (1953), 53–8

Meyer, T. *Geschichte des römischen Ärztestandes*. Kiel, 1907

Meyer-Steineg, T., *Das medizinische System der Methodiker*. Jena, 1916

Munzer, F., *Beiträge zur Quellenkritik der Naturgeschichte des Plinius*. Berlin, 1897

Orth, E., *Cicero und die Medizin*. Leipzig, 1925

Reiche, P., *Der Umfang der internmedizinischen Kenntnisse des Celsus*. Halle, 1934

Schmidt, A., *Drogen und Drogenhandel im Altertum*. Leipzig, 1924
'De origine apothecarum', *PIC⁶*, 108–11

Schouten, J., *The Rod and Serpent of Asklepios*. Amsterdam, 1967

Sévilla, H. J., 'L'art vétérinaire antique', *PIC³*, 274–87

Siegel, R. E., 'Galen's Experiments and Observations on Pulmonary Blood Flow and Respiration', *American Journal of Cardiology*, X (1962), 738–45
'The Influence of Galen's Doctrine of Pulmonary Bloodflow on the Development of Modern Concepts of Circulation', *AGM*, XLVI (1962), 311–32

Sigerist, H. E., 'The History of Medical Licensure', *Journal of the American Medical Association*, CIV (1935), 1057–60

Simboli, C. R., *Faith Cures in the Roman Empire in the First Two Centuries*. Diss., Columbia, 1919

Sinclair, T. A., 'Class Distinction in Medical Practice. A Piece of Ancient Evidence', *BHM*, XXV (1951), 386–7

Stannard, J., 'Materia Medica and Philosophic Theory in Aretaeus', *AGM*, XLVIII (1964), 27–53

Temkin, O. 'Epilepsy in an Anonymous Greek Work on Acute and Chronic Diseases', *BHM*, IV (1936), 137–44
The Falling Sickness. Baltimore, 1945
'Greek Medicine as Science and Craft', *Isis*, XLIV (1953), 213–25

Thévenot, E., 'Médecine et religion aux temps Gallo-Romains', *Latomus*, IX (1950), 415–26

van Andel, M. A., 'Folkmedical Themes in Myths, Legends, and Folktales', *PIC⁶*, 18–23

Veith, I., 'Galen's Psychology', *Perspectives in Biology and Medicine*, IV (1961), 316–23

Wellmann, M., 'A. Cornelius Celsus', *AGM*, XVI (1922), 289–313

Wilson, L. G., 'Erasistratus, Galen, and the Pneuma', *BHM*, XXXIII (1959), 293–314

Withington, E. T., 'Galen's Anatomy', *PIC³*, 96–100

INDEX